KT-226-123

Chest Pain
A man, a stent and a camper van

MICHAEL HARDING

HACHETTE
BOOKS
IRELAND

Copyright © 2019 Michael Harding

The right of Michael Harding to be identified as the Author of
the Work has been asserted by him in accordance with the
Copyright, Designs and Patents Act 1988.

First published in Ireland in 2019 by
HACHETTE BOOKS IRELAND

3

All rights reserved. No part of this publication may be reproduced,
stored in a retrieval system, or transmitted, in any form or by any means
without the prior written permission of the publisher, nor be otherwise
circulated in any form of binding or cover other than that in which
it is published and without a similar condition being imposed on the
subsequent purchaser.

'Sweet Killen Hill', a version of Peadar Ó Doirnín's poem,
by Tom MacIntyre, is reprinted by kind permission of Tom MacIntyre,
through the Jonathan Williams Literary Agency.
Extract from *Caisleáin Óir* by Seamus Ó Grianna used with permission of Mercier Press.

Some of the names and details within this text have been changed to
respect the privacy of individuals.

Cataloguing in Publication Data is available from the British Library

9781473690653

Typeset in Adobe Garamond Pro by www.grahamthew.com
Printed and bound in Great Britain by
Clays Ltd, Elcograf, S.p.A.

Hachette Books Ireland policy is to use papers that are natural, renewable
and recyclable products and made from wood grown in sustainable
forests. The logging and manufacturing processes are expected to
conform to the environmental regulations of the country of origin.

Hachette Books Ireland
8 Castlecourt Centre
Castleknock
Dublin 15, Ireland

A division of Hachette UK Ltd
Carmelite House, 50 Victoria Embankment, EC4Y 0DZ

www.hachettebooksireland.ie

PRAISE FOR MICHAEL HARDING

'Harding is a self-deprecating and winsome writer whose bittersweet musings on middle-age, loneliness and the search for spiritual enlightenment ... are leavened by an incredibly dry and unforced wit' *Metro Herald*

'Often funny, occasionally disturbing and not without its moments of deep sadness, Harding has peeled back his soul and held it out on the palm of his hand for all to see' Christine Dwyer-Hickey

'A repository of modern man's deepest fears, Harding emerges as something of an embattled hero for our times ... It's rare for a memoir to demand such intense emotional involvement, and rarer still for it to be so fully rewarded' *Sunday Times*

'Hilarious, and tender, and mad, and harrowing, and wistful, and always beautifully written. A wonderful book' Kevin Barry

'I read this book in one sitting ... Beautifully written ... *Staring at Lakes* gives us permission to be lost, sick, sad, creative, happy and compassionate – in short, to be human' Mary McEvoy, *Irish Independent*

'This memoir grabs you from the outset and holds you right to the end. His language sings' Deirdre Purcell

'Written in lyrical prose, it provides a compelling insight into the turbulent emotions that rage behind so many of the bland faces we meet in everyday life' *Sunday Business Post*

Windsor and Maidenhead

9580000126774

'This frank and unflinching memoir offers a fascinating insight into the mind of the author of two of the finest Irish novels of the eighties'
Pat McCabe

'Difficult to put down'
The Irish Times

Michael Harding is an author and playwright. His creative chronicle of ordinary life in the Irish midlands is published as a weekly column in *The Irish Times*. He has written numerous plays for the Abbey Theatre, including *Una Pooka*, *Misogynist* and *Sour Grapes*, and has published three novels, *Priest*, *The Trouble with Sarah Gullion* and *Bird in the Snow* as well as the award-winning, bestselling memoir *Staring at Lakes* (winner of the Bord Gais Energy Book of the Year), and *Hanging with the Elephant*, *Talking to Strangers* and *On Tuesdays I'm a Buddhist*.

For Cathy

Author's Note

Chest Pain is the memoir of a man, with a stent, and a camper van. Except that these remembrances are not complete historical records. It is not possible to portray the full complexity and riches of family life in any one book.

In each story I follow a single line, a strand of memory, and leave out much else.

All storytelling is an act of remembrance. But the art of memoir is a shaping of the past that allows us live more fully in the present.

I approach the past from different angles. Not just in each book but every day; every morning when I look in the mirror. Each day's memory is a fresh take on yesterday, which opens my heart a bit more into the present moment.

In 2018 I was so exhausted that I abandoned writing altogether; I closed my column in the *Irish Times*, and I struggled without success to write a book. I was fearful that I had come to the end of the road not just as a storyteller but as a human being.

Then the heart spoke, out of the blue, like the toll of a mighty bell, and almost immediately this book arrived, like a new beginning.

In previous books I have shared stories about mid-life depression (*Staring at Lakes*), the loss of mother (*Hanging with the Elephant*), the search for identity (*Talking to Strangers*), and the struggle with various forms of therapy (*On Tuesdays I'm a Buddhist*).

Lying in a coronary care unit became the start of an entirely new chapter. The beginning of looking at everything in a new light.

The one constant in my life has been the joy of a family and the company of the beloved.

But there is a part in all of us that exists only in solitude. An inner self that never surfaces in the light of day. A self that exists beyond thoughts or emotions and cannot be defined by relationships. A singularity almost beyond any existing self that can only be described in poetic language.

In the deepest recesses of my heart there exists a kind of mythic figure, like a monk in his cave.

'He is the self that watches your self,' as my therapist used to say.

And telling his story is an act so private and personal that it feels like beginning all over again.

Some of the names and details within this text have been changed.

Contents

THE JIGS

The rude awakening • 3

The greasy sausages • 11

Orange marigolds • 15

Every little detail • 23

The guard in the supermarket aisle • 39

Seven brass bowls • 47

Tiers of a wedding cake • 55

The shiny black bonnet • 63

Fake beauty • 69

A fine May morning • 73

The same as before • 77

THE REELS

A new pair of togs • 85

The track bottoms • 93

Golden castles • 103

Spoons from yesterday • 111

The angel and the fish • 119

Five nuns • 125

The remembrance reel • 137

Round glasses with a wide bridge • 153

The Irish snowstorm • 165

OLD HORNPIPES
The fish in the fridge • 173
Coming off the fence • 177
The cup of tea with toast • 181
Paper lanterns • 187
The far away hornpipe • 193
The baby in the pram • 197
Accidental events • 201
Dreaming of clocks • 215
Accidents in the afternoon • 221
Grief poured out • 225
Footsteps • 229
Begin again • 233

THE SLOW AIRS OF THE MOUNTAIN
Completing a miracle • 251
The death of strangers • 263
Snow • 267
Poached eggs • 275
The virgin in the crib • 279
The white-haired man • 283
Enjoy yourself, it's later than you think • 295
Fish and chips, and the takeaway van • 301

Acknowledgements • 309

THE JIGS

The rude awakening

I thought I was capable of loving, but maybe I made a mistake, because sometimes a man can talk the talk, but forever walk alone. And when I look back on sixty-five years of life, I admit that I talked a lot, and I cried and sang about love and tenderness. But when it came to walking the walk I was often, in my own little way, a very solitary person.

I may have written about being a man in the modern world, and I may have spoken about God, and Mother, and human longing, but did I really know how much my own heart mattered?

Writers talk a lot and are full of ideas; but sometimes the feelings and emotions are forgotten.

Perhaps I did not even know how to open my heart fully to the world, until I had a heart attack.

At least that's how I felt, as I sat in the lounge of the Abbey Hotel in Roscommon at the end of May 2019, listening to such a beautiful conversation at the next table; where every single word the young couple spoke flowed from heart to heart, and every spoken word embodied love; fumbled, muttered, whispered, but all uttered in trembling affection for one another. It felt like the very rafters of the hotel might be shivering with emotion at the sound of their voices.

And I was happy too, at my table, planning a camping trip to Donegal which would bring me back to the long white beaches I once relished as a boy, and to the coastline around which my beloved and I had cycled in 1987.

The couple at the next table were planning their wedding, and they exuded such warmth and excitement as they pored over the details that I felt a mixture of joy for their future and sorrow for the shortness of any life, all in a single moment.

The lounge of the Abbey Hotel was as intimate as a large drawing room. It was noon, and I was enjoying the sunshine of another bright day in May. On a distant radio the Angelus bell tolled its final ring for noon. I was passing the time until 3 p.m. when I hoped to collect the camper van in Ballyfarnon from Frank Healy's garage. Frank was replacing a headlamp, an indicator bulb on the passenger side and a pulley for the alternator. He was putting on two new tyres because, when I bought the van two weeks earlier up in Donegal, the rear tyres were badly frayed and one was slowly leaking air.

Of course Frank would also change the oil, and put in new filters. He was an excellent mechanic and I trusted him totally. I had relied on him for years. I had no worry when I handed over money for the van and saw the 03 number plates and the clock showing 140,000 miles. I might not know much about

4

what was under the bonnet, but I was certain that everything would get a thorough inspection later on, from Frank. So I didn't dally. I bought the van on the spot.

And now the day was almost upon us. On the morrow the van would be ready for its maiden voyage. I would drive away from our house in the hills above Lough Allen and up through Manorhamilton, onwards through the Leitrim glens, towards the hills and beaches of Donegal. It was an adventure I had been promising myself for six months, ever since I ended up in a hospital bed not far from Blanchardstown shopping centre in early December 2018.

As I came into the hotel that morning I could smell beef from a carvery counter. And I hoped it might be open. I stood in the archway sniffing the gravy as a dark-haired woman appeared behind the counter with a long tray of salmon cutlets and slipped them into position beside the beef.

'Am I too early for lunch?' I wondered.

'You're too early for a lot of things,' she said, smiling.

'OK,' I replied. 'So could you give me a coffee?'

She stared at me for a second and then smiled more.

'I know that voice,' she declared.

And I guessed she recognised me from the television. Maybe *The Late Late Show* or *The Ray D'Arcy Show*, which I often appeared on anytime I had a book on the market.

'I can give you whatever you want,' she said, 'so long as I can have a photograph with you for my husband. He's mad about you. Every time you come on the television he's jumping up to record it.'

So I stood beside her, and she got a young chef from the kitchen, a gangly teenage boy with red hair, wearing a white uniform and a white hat, to come out and take the picture. He scrutinised me for a moment as if he hoped I might be some famous singer; but I wasn't. And when he didn't recognise me his face dropped. Clearly, for him I was a huge disappointment. Anyway, he took the picture, and then I sat in the lounge and the waitress went off and got me an Americano.

6   That's when I noticed the couple near the window. They were talking to the manager about the banquet for their upcoming wedding.

The sun was shining outside the window and a breeze was tossing big chestnut branches into a flustery dance of luminous green leaf.

My heart attack, though it had happened only six months earlier, felt remote. I pushed it away as if it had happened centuries ago.

Although it had left it's mark. My legs still felt like they were made of lead, and sometimes I got twinges or needles of pain in my chest, and every day I took six tablets. And I knew I had only just escaped catastrophe.

I became watery-eyed with joy when the sun broke through the clouds, and shafts of dazzling light seeped in through the hotel window.

If a heart attack is akin to an earthquake, then the epicentre might be located at the moment in time when the event took place, the very second that the imaginary bus hit the chest. For me that moment arrived at a few minutes past 9 a.m. on Saturday, 8 December 2018. From that zero hour, the shockwaves seeped out, in both directions, both forwards and backwards in time, changing the way I had viewed the past, and saturating my perceptions of life to come with little question marks.

As the waves of shock rippled through me, my memories altered; I reinterpreted things differently. My future appeared more fragile. And all my assumptions about robust health and expectations of a long life were shattered. I had thought about death all my life to the point of obsession. But now I felt it.

It was a rude awakening, a minor enlightenment more profound than anything I had ever experienced as a result of practising religion or studying philosophy.

When the coronary event occurred, everything about my life began to feel like straw, and I began to understand a few essential truths that all religions teach.

Life is passing, and it is over in a flash, and the only place to find the kingdom of heaven is in the present moment. And there are no teachings in any tradition worth so much as an aspirin.

I suppose that's as much enlightenment as anyone could hope for.

I fell against the wall of an underground car park on a Wednesday three days before the attack, but I suspected that the cause was stress. I fell against the railings on the promenade in Bray on Friday, the day before the event, but I thought that was indigestion.

I soldiered on and I could hardly walk back to my hotel in Blanchardstown after being on stage on Friday evening but I blamed exhaustion. And then at nine o'clock on Saturday, the following morning, my heart flipped into a tizzy of irregular palpitations. I just couldn't push the blood through the clogged arteries any longer. I began to feel the beats like hammer blows on an anvil, deep inside my ribcage.

The struggle might have ended in a massive inward convulsion killing me instantly or within half an hour, had it not been for the good fortune that I was in a hotel in Blanchardstown. But there's no doubt that in those critical moments while I waited for the ambulance, the bursting heart was a ruthless teacher.

So in the wake of that event I vowed to change my life. I solemnly promised to avoid stress, excessive amounts of drink, endless hours on the couch watching television, and to eat fewer buns full of raisins with my lattes.

The camper van was a strategy. It would change everything; it would become a magical wishing jewel, to transform my universe. It would become like the chalice I once received on the day I was ordained a priest; that same chalice I finally tried to dispose of on the top of Skellig Michael in the summer of 2017, although in the end I couldn't bear to be parted from it.

The camper van would be no different from the water bowls I got from a monk in India in 1995. And it would be like the old typewriter my uncle gave me in 1968. Because all those objects, typewriter, chalice and water bowls, were instruments of transformation.

And the camper van would be no less. Another magical jewel in my romantic narrative. Another source of blessing for my naive heart.

Only a few years earlier I had fallen into the trap of magical thinking with an icon my beloved brought home from Poland. Another person might have hung it on the wall and seen it as an art object. But I spent a year gazing at it and imagining that it was gazing back at me.

9

The universe was always a magical place for me, and magical thinking was the only response. The typewriter turned me into a writer. The chalice turned me into a priest. The water bowls taught me how to meditate and find calm abiding even in the storms of depression. And as I lay in hospital on a winter's morning at the end of 2018, with a new stent, a long but tiny cylinder lodged inside an artery on the left of my heart muscle, which allowed the blood to flow like it never flowed before, I had my first vision of a camper van. It rose before me like a gleaming chariot that would take me out of danger.

The very thought of it cheered me and my heart purred like a Mercedes-Benz engine as I rested in the surgical room of the Mater Private, after the procedure.

My heart beat with the rhythm of the ocean. I had not died. I had escaped the worst possibility, due to the early intervention of paramedics. And I had been given another chance at life, to live a little longer and to say yes to the cosmos; and yes to a camper van.

The greasy sausages

In the autumn of 2018 I'd toured Ireland, doing readings from my books at arts centres, town halls and in other community centres. By the first week in December I'd had only five gigs left. It had been a long road, from Tralee to Letterkenny, and Carrickmacross to Wexford through twenty-eight venues. The only calamity was when my radio microphone went dead one night on stage in Bray, even though I had bought a new battery for the headset that afternoon. But it only took me a few seconds to replace it, and I was back in business, sharing stories about life as a bewildered male, and how I cope with the absurdity of old age.

I was tired as I walked off stage that night and I didn't sleep well, so the next morning I treated myself to a full Irish breakfast, and I went for a walk on Bray's seafront promenade. I was only at the beginning of the walk when pain between my shoulder blades lashed me to the railings, and I was forced to shuffle back to the car.

Maybe I should have resisted those big sausages, I mused,

remembering the breakfast. Because I was clearly suffering from indigestion.

I was due on stage in Blanchardstown that evening so I headed up the M50 towards Exit 6. All around the Blanchardstown Centre early-morning shoppers were already stuffing gift parcels and shopping bags into the rear ends of a thousand cars in the parking lots in anticipation of Christmas, three weeks away.

I checked into a hotel nearby and went to my room on the seventh floor, where I stood at the window looking out. Far below me the traffic moved around the square, bumper to bumper, brake lights twinkling in the mid-winter morning beyond the curtained windows. I lay on the bed for most of the afternoon.

In the theatre that evening the technical manager said, 'You look tired,' as we sound-checked the microphone.

I said, 'It's been a long tour.'

I had a coffee and a KitKat in the dressing room, as I stared into the mirror and waited for eight o'clock.

I had no pain on stage. But as soon as the show was over, and even before I returned to the dressing room, a muffled knot of stiff muscle crept across my chest, up my neck and down my arms.

All I could think of was that breakfast: rashers and eggs, black pudding and three big sausages.

'I definitely should have skipped the sausages,' I muttered.

Because I presumed my heart was in excellent condition. I

had spent years walking around the hills above Lough Allen. I had given up cigarettes when I was forty. I had walked the pilgrim path across Sliabh Liag in Donegal twice, and endured the freezing fog of Warsaw streets on many winter nights. So how could there be anything wrong with my heart?

In my hotel bedroom the pain persisted, so I phoned the beloved. I should have asked her did she know anything about heart attacks, but I didn't want to worry her. Just like I didn't want to worry her the previous year when I noticed I couldn't walk up hills as easily as I used to. Just as I didn't want to worry her when I realised that swimming half a length of the pool was leaving me breathless. In fact it wasn't any concern for her that caused me to hide my weakening health. It was the horror of appearing vulnerable that kept my mouth shut.

'There's something wrong,' she said. 'What is it?'

'Indigestion,' I suggested.

My heart, like a caged bird, was screaming for attention. But I talked about sausages.

After the phone call I lay awake in the dark.

It didn't feel like a blacksmith's hammer beating the anvil any longer. It felt like a blacksmith's horse stepping on and off my ribcage. Although when I manoeuvred my body into different positions, the pain went away. And eventually I fell asleep.

I woke at 7 a.m. It was still dark. But the pain kept returning with the regularity of ocean waves.

'Big greasy sausages,' I hissed. 'Never again.'

13

I reached for the laptop and googled 'indigestion'. It was my final act of denial.

From the bottomless well of learning that exists on the internet, Doctor Google assembled for me an array of reassuring possibilities. For example, if I stretched my neck in different directions, the indigestion would dissipate.

So he said. And so I did.

And sure enough the pain diminished. Clearly the problem was, indeed, indigestion. A few exercises should cure it.

Tai chi is very good in these situations, Doctor Google added.

And having lost all ability at rational thought, on the seventh floor of a four-star hotel I stood pot-bellied in my pyjamas and began leaping through half-remembered tai chi movements, like a Taoist master drowning in quicksand, or like a duck trying to dance the lead in *Swan Lake*.

And the pain dissolved.

'There you go!' I exclaimed triumphantly at the mirror. 'It's gone. Nothing to worry about!'

But then it returned. This time a pain like the front of a bus impacting on my chest at high speed, a pain bigger than my body was capable of sustaining. And I knew, beyond all shadow of doubt or delusion, that I was having what even Doctor Google would describe as an acute heart attack. I phoned for help. And because I was so close to the hospital, the emergency team arrived in under ten minutes. They got tablets into me just in time. Another few minutes and it might have been too late.

14

Orange marigolds

My beloved wife arrived into the hotel room at the same moment as the paramedics. She had come from Leitrim. All through the night and during the previous day I had lied to her on the phone.

I said I was fine. There was nothing to worry about. The pain in my chest wasn't actually a pain. And it wasn't actually in the chest. It was in the neck. And no, I had no intention of getting into a taxi and driving to a hospital, as she urged me to do at one point, just before midnight.

'Think of what a taxi might cost,' I barked. 'Think of what it would be like in an emergency room for hours on a trolley, with everyone looking at me, half naked, like an old man.'

I didn't want to be caught in that kind of situation. An old man on a trolley is as vulnerable as a child in a cot, and often more terrified. But shame prevented me even contemplating the naked vulnerability of old age, never mind sharing my anxieties with the beloved.

I had not been honest with either myself or the beloved about my deteriorating health, which was particularly odd because I was a writer.

You'd expect a writer to tell someone how they felt. But I just wrote things down. Writing allowed me avoid having to tell the truth, face to face. But by March of 2018, even the writing had stopped. I closed down my weekly column in *The Irish Times*. Some unconscious instinct that the final solitude of death was close at hand kept gnawing at me. I couldn't name it but I felt that the word processor should be silenced.

16   And there was another issue. Another big secret. Another solitude. And another betrayal.

Prayer is not a fashionable word, and sometimes I feel ashamed that I spent so much time exploring not one but two religious traditions with all their attendant misogynies and intellectual bluff. I had been a Catholic priest and a student of Tibetan Buddhism. But the one constant for me was the act of prayer, the faltering attempt to greet the mystery of life with the heart rather than the brain.

I was ordained a priest in 1981. Almost forty years later the chalice still sat on my shelf of holy objects. The photographs were still resting in an album in some drawer of memorabilia. And though I fled from that dry clerical life when I was thirty-one, I began again at forty, on another long journey into silence, by taking refuge with all my heart in the Panchen Ötrul Rinpoche, distinguished lama in the Gelugpa school of Tibetan philosophy.

How to balance a spiritual path with a happy marriage wasn't easy, but I tried. The walls of my studio gradually filled up with Buddhas and thankas over the years. But when a Christian icon appeared on my desk in 2016, as a gift from the beloved, I found myself turning again to the Mother of God and the Holy Christ for occasional consolation. Stirring bits of this and bits of that into a single pot, I made a soup of my devotions.

And I remember the nuns from Minsk, those strait-laced Orthodox sisters from the Saint Elisabeth Convent in Belarus, being appalled one day when they came into the studio. They had made a few attempts to visit us previously without success, but when they finally arrived on the doorstep and came into my workspace their faces turned as white as a bucket of milk as they gazed at so many holy faces from diverse religious traditions staring back at them from every wall. They were horrified.

From Padre Pio and the Mother of Jesus to Buddha Manjushri and the Lady Buddha Tara, my walls were a veritable gallery of religiosity, a fusion of two belief systems that had been blended over the years from the mix and remix of my eclectic spiritual preferences.

But I was comfortable in my multi-denominational man cave. It was other people I felt were a threat.

Call it man cave or studio, it was where I prayed. And nobody could interfere or undermine that. Especially since I didn't flaunt my devotions. I privatised faith, believing that was the only acceptable way to go, considering all the damage religion had done to women and children as a public institution. But it didn't occur to me that hiding away from people in my room was itself a manifestation of misogyny, an example of the very guff I complained about in others.

I didn't realise how solitude in itself can be the foundation of men's misogynies. Even in marriage, privacy can be a tyranny that undermines intimacy until autonomy becomes cancerous and begins to eat away at everything.

The intimacy of family life often appeared like a threat to my serenity.

18   But all that masculinity came crashing down when one slippery heartbeat faltered. When one big bus in the chest challenged the autonomy and the sovereignty of my self.

The men around me in the coronary care unit were in similar states of shock; our bodies rested in the afternoons, accommodating our arteries to the shining new stents. I could almost hear the blood flowing everywhere more freely. And I could see it in their faces, the same bewilderment as in my own.

I wondered how I could have been so proud, and kept my beloved at arm's length for so long; she was the one who loved me most, and whose love might have undercut all that blather from Doctor Google. And how many other times, I wondered, had I betrayed her without realising it?

And I was still wondering, on that bright May day in 2019.

That's when I noticed the couple at the next table as they talked to the manager about their wedding.

They discussed the size of their cake and how many tiers it ought to have. And my heart was breaking to think of it. And to think how far a couple can travel from the first beginnings of love to the complexity of its final closure; writing wills, and making sure the world is legally tidy for the children when it's all over.

I remember when I used to get carnal urges just mowing the lawn. The smell of grass intoxicated me. The smell of the barbecue sent my libido into meltdown, and wine was like petrol poured on a fire of hot, melting lust, especially at midsummer parties that went on all night while house guests stretched like cats behind cream curtains. And if we did go to bed, it was only to lie awake listening to the pheasants and make love to a backdrop of birdsong as the sun came up.

But time passes. A man grows old. And eventually we were forced to fly off to exotic places like Faro in Portugal to stir the libido with heat and sunbeds and tequilas beside the pool.

Portugal had been the last straw. I'd vowed it would be my final sun holiday. The last time, I'd promised myself, that I would ever seek pleasure in a world that had no meaning beyond the act of lathering the body with suntan lotion, or the pernickety obsessive rituals of trying exotic foods and drinks in the late evening. I'd seen one too many crispy-fleshed elders make their way to and from their sunbeds at the pool, their skin sizzling like rashers beneath the buttery suntan oil.

I used to seek out old churches in order to sit in the shade and keep cool, and maybe that's what began the gradual re-awakening of my religious fervour. It was around the turn of the millennium. And I remember one morning when we came home, I found nuts in the old shed at the back of the house and I wasn't sure where they came from. They might have been stones from the cherry tree, brought there and cracked open by birds. Or a rogue squirrel, occupying the shed over a few harsh winters. And the pine marten and the hawfinch had also been accused. The beloved had a theory that the stones were from plums, not cherries at all. And the old shed began to sound like a protected habitat for exotic animals. So it made for a dizzy debate in the kitchen, because even then, when we had returned from that sun holiday, I wanted to dismantle the shed and put up a new building as soon as I could. I wanted a refuge from the world even though the studio wasn't finally built until 2012.

We designed it with a patio door facing the lake, and no window looking towards the house. It was perfect for a writer. Turned away from the home, it was a place apart, with its own separate gate, where I could sit all day if I wanted, reading poetry or filling little Tibetan water bowls to the brim.

Even if the lady wife was indoors with neighbours drinking green tea, and discussing the merits of brewing orange marigolds, as they were wont to do in those years, I could remain aloof in my solitary den and look at the water.

I had always been romantic about solitude. The sculptor shaving dust from stone with a chisel or the monk doodling on cowhide were to me examples of how beauty grew in solitary contemplation.

Four years ministering as a priest had taught me that celibacy was a public posture; it was an affirmation of chastity and a refusal of intimacy, and it was undertaken for the sake of a heavenly realm. For the celibate, there was no point in embracing any other, because whatever human love was, it couldn't last. To remain alone was a sign that we were all destined for elsewhere; somewhere further up the road called heaven. Celibacy was a kind of public posturing – the coat-trailing, flag-waving embodiment of a sexless life.

Solitude, on the other hand, was different from celibacy. Solitude was the real thing. It was a private affair of the heart, and rather than asserting splendid isolation like the celibate cleric in a car of his own, solitude was a monastic virtue lived out in community.

When monks practised solitude, they did it quietly, and together. The intimacy of monastic life was not unlike a family. In solitude a person could become conscious, awake, enlightened, and more easily able to embrace others, rather than just living without them.

Which begs the question I can't answer: what drew me to celibacy?

And what drew me to other religious traditions? What enchanted me about icons and sacred objects, and what created in me the delusion that I was not alone when I was alone?

I still don't have any answers.

All I know is that in 2018 my Christian faith returned again like an old virus. Or like a fire that made me breathless, so that I couldn't walk up a hill without getting exhausted.

Every little detail

How sweet my coffee was, at the end of May, in the Abbey Hotel in Roscommon town. The couple close to me went over every detail in their notes with the manager. They had scribbled their ideas on the back of a large envelope overnight and now they were going through them and 'leaving no stone unturned', as the manager put it.

As if their love was so vast that they needed to weave an enormous tapestry of ritual and commitment in public, just to express it. As if all the cakes and red carpets, the candles and scented flowers, were only threads to hold together the enormity of their vows.

A wedding is not just about joining hands, or pressing lips to another person's fingers, or gazing in awe at the bands of gold lying on the silver dish. Those are only the private bits.

But this was a public thing. And every little detail mattered.

It was about how they might smile into the camera. What type of coverings would go on the seats at the banquet. Where would the priest sit?

Every commitment to detail was an intricate expression of love. And even the price of providing a meal for so many guests was as naught compared to the devotion they intended to offer each other in that elaborate ritual of 'their wedding day'.

I was almost in tears as I listened, and munched a biscuit and sipped an Americano and waited for the carvery lunch counter to open.

I wanted to turn around and say to them, 'Do you realise you are beginning the greatest adventure of your life? And even though I am sitting here in the same lounge, thinking only of my stomach, I am excited for you. Because I have stood where you are standing now.'

Many years ago I'd promised my beloved the sun, moon and stars. And then I'd failed, and failed again.

We'd both failed.

Because as life is lived out, the promises turn out to be less than was dreamed of.

But a couple endures, and hold to the promise. And even promise more. And live more. Always reaching, and always failing. Always deepening in love through every failure.

If I were still a priest, I would stand before them and give a sermon so long that they'd be pleading with me to shut up.

'Each time you fail,' I would say, 'you will begin again. Because you made a promise. You take your life up in your hands, like water, on this your wedding day, and it will run through your fingers so many times, and so many times you will lose it; but you will gather it out of the well again and again. Marriage is not just haphazard joy, but the living out of an intention. Each new day has been already promised, each to each. Each morning is his gift to you and yours to him. It's not the tragedies or grief you pass through that will shape you, but this promise, with which you endure such tragedies. The promise of love for each other.

'The act of love and the rituals of intimacy are not just casual moments of pleasure or spontaneous generosity; they are the fulfilment of all the promise you hold in your hands on your wedding day.'

25

'Dear Jesus,' I whispered into my Americano, 'if only I could have walked the walk as well as just this talking talk.'

And no, I wouldn't like to be the priest at their wedding. To be celibate at a wedding would be for me no less terrible than to be blind in Granada.

'Let me tell you about the speeches,' the manager said. 'There are a few issues you need to be aware of. Firstly, you want to have speeches after the food. Is that correct?'

'Yes. That's what we want,' the groom replied. 'That's the best.'

'Good. Because if you have the speeches before the food then you don't know how long that will take, and the food will go cold.'

The bride didn't like this idea.

'I'd definitely like them at the beginning, and get them over with,' she said. 'Then we can enjoy the meal.'

'I hear you,' the manager said, 'but at least have a think about it.'

The bride explained that she might be nervous. That she wanted to give a speech, but that she would be sick and wouldn't eat if she was waiting until after the desserts.

'OK. Well, maybe have one speech beforehand,' the manager suggested. 'Let the bride speak and then have the other speeches afterwards.'

When myself and the beloved had decided to marry we'd asked a friend, Pat O'Brien, who was a curate in Skehana, County Galway, to do some kind of service for us. It had begun as a small idea. A little blessing, perhaps. But it had turned into a full wedding.

It was a windswept day in the middle of April, 1993. The bride's brothers and sisters came. My mother looked dainty in a little blue suit. The bride's son looked elegant in a white shirt and waistcoat, his long hair flowing over his shoulders.

'Who's that?' my mother wanted to know.

'That's my new stepson,' I declared cheerfully.

'Right,' she said, and she danced with him later at the house party.

A few people turned out in white hats. After the service was over they all walked down the road to Costello's Bar for drinks, a country pub with a green galvanised roof and a latch on the door and a pot-bellied stove on the concrete floor.

They drank to love, and joy, and recklessness, and someone sang 'Caledonia', and then the bride and I drove off in a little mini car, with cans attached by pink ribbons to the back bumper, and everyone followed us up through the winding roads of Roscommon, Tulsk, Elphin and Carrick-on-Shannon, to the outskirts of a village called Keadue, where we planned to begin our new life in a rented farmhouse hidden in birch woods and bogland away from any main road.

Friends of the beloved made cakes and cooked rice and pasta dishes that were set out on a table in the garden, and we had seventeen litres of wine in boxes that we bought the previous week in Enniskillen.

Friends on guitars and accordions provided music, and as the sun went down people danced inside and outside the house, in the kitchen and on the lawn. The cake was displayed on a stone wall at the end of the garden so that everyone could see myself and the beloved cut it in slices.

I thanked people for coming. I claimed her as the love of my life. And I quoted lines from Tom MacIntyre's version of the Peadar Ó Doirnín poem 'Sweet Killen Hill'.

Flower of the flock,
Any time, any land,
Plenty your ringlets,
Plenty your hand,
Sunlight your window,
Laughter your sill,

And I must be with you
On sweet Killen Hill.
...
Gentle one, lovely one,
Come to me,
Now sleep the clergy,
Now sleep their care,
Sunrise will find us
But sunrise won't tell
That love lacks surveillance
On sweet Killen Hill.

And so it was. And the celebrations went on all night, and a bonfire was lit in the field, and at dawn I ascended the stairs to her bedroom where she was already asleep and I lay beside her, awake and in trepidation about our future.

I tried to make sense of this marriage. The day had passed as if I was in a play. I played the role of the groom. But I wasn't in control. And all the guests were merely actors in the ritual: mothers and fathers, old friends and distant relations.

But the centre of it all was her. And it was official now. She was my beloved, from this day forth. And in the ritual of the day, she was the queen of everything. And I was her Duke of Edinburgh.

That is how I felt, lying awake beside her, a husband on the threshold, and trembling.

My life had changed. I could not continue in the old dispensation. In the kingdom of me. And even though she slept soundly and her breath rose and fell like the ocean, it impelled me. Her presence created in me an imperative; she was calling me away from self-obsession.

And yet paradoxically, to be of any use to her, I felt I should go even deeper into the silent world that men call the inner room of the heart.

Because without standing on my own ground, in silence, how could I be fit to stand beside her.

That is the conundrum of the solitary life. It's a betrayal of the beloved, and yet, without it, there is nothing to offer the beloved other than a stick banging an empty drum.

'I go out to you,' I whispered. 'I go out not knowing where this will end, or in what tears.' That was my real speech at the wedding, whispered at her sleeping body early in the morning. And I knew it would always be this way, a promise made but never quite fulfilled.

'I will weave my solitude around yours,' I whispered at her sleeping figure, 'until we are both grey-haired and silent, in our separate armchairs, with no more need to speak.'

It was a promise.

'And no matter how many small deceits creep into our marriage from time to time, this will be the place to which we will always return.'

I was glad she slept and didn't hear such sentimental drivel in the middle of the night.

The manager and the young couple talked on about their own issues. The manager was still pursuing speeches after the meal and not, as the bride wanted, before.

'Of course it's up to you,' the manager said. 'I'd just advise you to wait until afterwards. Because I know what the outcome will be. Because we do it every week. And the chef knows what works and what doesn't work when he's trying to hold up the food and keep things warm in the oven for hundreds of people.'

They were having three hundred guests.

30 'Well, you're looking at forty minutes while they are coming into the hotel, hanging around the bar and the foyer. Then they freshen up in the bathrooms. And then we call everyone into the function room. We will have taken their orders of course before they come in.'

The bride was smiling now, visualising all this great ritual and where she might stand in her white gown with all its ruffles and veils waiting for the bell to ring for dinner.

'Will I be OK' she wondered, 'in my gown? Like, will I be just standing around?'

'Oh,' the manager said, 'you won't be just standing around. You'll be the bride!'

And the idea of total transformation began to hit the young woman and I saw her face flushing now as she listened.

Yes, I thought to myself. Yes, you'll be fine. You can see the future now. This wedding is going to be huge. It will shape everything.

'So let's talk about time,' the manager said. 'I can advise you that maybe 5 p.m. is good. But not later than 5.15. It gives you a chance to chat to people and relax with your friends.

'And even when we have rung the bell you can still have that forty minutes to chat. And you're looking at sitting down for 6 p.m. And then 8.30 p.m. or 9 p.m. your band starts. And I know you paid big money for the band so you want to get them going.'

The couple held hands. They were emotionally exhausted just going through the various stages of the big day.

The manager noticed it. 'Don't worry,' she said, 'I'll go over all this again later. Closer to the day.

'But,' she warned them, 'it's the knock-on effect you have to watch out for: 4.15 p.m. for the photographer. And you need to avoid delays. So the bell goes at 5.15 p.m. And at 6 p.m. we're sitting down and ready to go with the food.'

'Will there be a red carpet?' the bride wondered.

'Oh yes,' the groom said, taking a little manly control, 'we definitely want a red carpet.'

'So that's no problem,' the manager said. 'You have the platinum package. That covers the red carpet and the sparkling wine and summer punch when people are arriving. And sandwiches, tea and coffee at the end.'

'Can we have sandwiches at the beginning as well?'

'If you like. Certainly. But would you not prefer just something for yourself? When you arrive?'

'No,' the bride said adamantly.

'Are you sure?' her beloved wondered.

She was certain. 'But the people should have a drink when they arrive. Mammy is in her seventies.'

She was thinking selflessly already. I suppose it's almost impossible to give yourself to another person in some ritual of religious dimensions and not submit to the fantasy of self-annihilation.

The manager didn't think that a drink for everybody on arrival was necessary.

'Look, basically you can have bottles of Prosecco,' she said, 'but that's extra money. And you don't really need them if people are going to the bar buying their own drinks. Which is probably what most people do.'

'OK,' the bride murmured. 'OK. That's OK.'

I suppose when young people start out they know as little about marriage as they do about pension funds. The future is not relevant. Their expectation is for happiness, the soft cocoon that they imagine marriage will be. They don't realise that the partnership provides meaning in life rather than happiness. When you fall in love, marriage has the potential to give life a shape and context. You make the promise, and even if it doesn't work out, your entire life has been shaped by the event. And life changes people too – illness, death, flawed sex, imperfect children and financial disasters. You can never anticipate what will happen. You can only surf the future like a wave when it arrives and hold onto the promise that was made so public at the beginning: I will share this with you.

When I see young people of differing sexes or the same sex preparing for their wedding day I gush with emotion and am grateful that I too enjoyed such a moment, even if, as everybody now knows, marriage long ago may have been a licence for abuse, a kingdom of the patriarch or a room of slavery for disempowered women.

I remember an old woman in Mullingar who was frightened by a gramophone. It wasn't right to have a man singing in a box inside her house, she said. I never heard her reflect much on whether or not marriage was a good idea, but at least she delighted in her son Tommy, who had a musical ear.

'He was only a child standing in the cot when he could play "The Rose of Aranmore" on the accordion,' she told me proudly.

And when she herself was young she got fourpence for half a dozen eggs, and a pound of sugar cost fourpence, so she'd stand for days waiting for eggs to drop from the hen's arse, dreaming of sugar.

'That's what marriage was about in our day,' she said. 'From the time I walked down the aisle at seventeen years of age there was nothing soft about it. Nothing romantic.'

She had white hair and she made tea and we ate warm bread in her kitchen.

'Did men ever frighten you?' I wondered.

'Only Germans,' she said. 'I was terrified in case they'd come as far as Mullingar. There was a big house near here with a thousand-acre field and they put stakes in the field so that planes wouldn't be able to land.'

'Were there any tragedies in your family?' I wondered.

'There were no inhalers for the bad chest,' she replied. 'And the forge was dirty and there was a fire in the middle of it under a thatched roof and the straws hanging down were black with soot. And when the war came we used anthracite. So the straws turned white, and me uncle was inhaling it until it killed him.'

She remembered her brother being born all of a sudden, and the handywoman coming and her hands not washed.

'I fetched the buckets of water,' she said, 'to wash the child and make the tea. And later the council appointed a nurse for the district and the handywomen weren't needed after that.'

'Were you happy in marriage?' I asked.

Her face darkened.

'Marriage at that time was a dangerous business,' she said. 'I seen a woman go into labour and she was at it from a Monday morning to the following Sunday when the baby come, dead, at ten pounds weight. And then the following morning the mother died. She was thirty-nine. You wouldn't leave a cow in labour that long. A full week and a clot in her neck finished her, and when she died there was a big black mark all down her neck. I remember it as if it were yesterday. And that's what marriage meant in our day. But if you had your husband you had someone to share it with. We both knew that. Sure who else did you have except your man?'

'But,' I wondered, 'what if you didn't share your feelings?'

The old woman scrutinised my face. 'What do you mean?' she asked. She didn't understand the question. 'Why wouldn't you share your feelings?' she wondered, and she didn't expect an answer.

In the 1980s before we married, my beloved and I would spend wintry afternoons in a Dublin cinema, watching the screen through a plume of smoke. Sometimes to avoid distracting other punters with my cigarette lighter, I would light a fresh cigarette from the beloved's. Butt to cigarette butt was like a ritual kiss, sucking fire from one to the other, in a gesture of delicate intimacy.

We didn't care what damage cigarettes might do because we didn't live in the future. Love back then was a cocoon of the present moment, fortified and endurable and big enough for two. And at least we were having more fun than our grandparents. Or so we thought.

In the late 1990s, we went away for a night to celebrate our anniversary in a Galway hotel. In the middle of the night I wanted to go to the bathroom. My mind was floating in the lake of a dream. Only my body rose from the sheets.

The path was automatic. Marriage is a series of habitual motions, and the bathroom was not difficult to find in our little cottage. Except that I was not at home so when my eyes eventually opened, consciousness surfaced like a giant eel in Lough Allen, and I found myself standing in the corridor, in the middle of the night, dressed only in my pyjama top.

The door of the room was only three feet away but it was locked. My only hope was to knock and pray that the companion of my life would not let me down. Would not sleep on through the moment of my tribulation in the top of a pyjamas on the second floor of a luxurious hotel.

But she didn't wake.

I tried harder. A sharper tapping on the door. A rapping on the door. I was panicking. A strong, persistent incantation of her name. What a wonderful sleeper she was.

Then someone did wake and a door opened. Not ours, but the one across the corridor, and a very cross lady in a dressing gown examined me from the rear.

'I suppose you're happy now,' she said. 'You've got everyone awake.' And she slammed the door.

But I was still stuck. And I could hear snoring sounds from all the other lovely rooms. I could hear whispering and giggling and television stations, and muffled sounds of happy punters who had paid their money for the night of luxury.

But not me. I was on the outside and my wife, by sleeping so heavily, had betrayed me.

I tied the pyjama top around my waist like a skirt, and headed down the corridor in search of the lift.

To my relief the reception area was empty. Distant voices of the night staff floated from the kitchen, where they were enjoying their midnight dinner. I sneaked in behind the reception desk, got the phone and dialled room 1003.

Her voice was like salvation. Her voice was like the music of the heavens.

How I love this woman, I thought. I need her so much. I depend on her.

'It's me,' I said. 'I locked myself out. Can you open the door?'

There was a long pause.

'Who's this?' she asked.

'It's me,' I said. 'It's fucking me.'

The most existential declaration of identity I had ever known.

'It's me,' I said. And it was. Me. Hiding under the reception desk of a Galway hotel. But it was us, later, in the cosy bed, after a big bath, all night long and lots of food and drink. That was us.

It's me, I had said, naked and frightened, underneath the reception desk. Hoping she would claim to know me, and open the door.

In the bath it was not me, but us. A couple. Married. Going forward.

The guard in the supermarket aisle

I have no privacy in supermarkets. I can't hide who I am when people are browsing the contents of my basket.

Recently I was walking around a supermarket trying to remember what I came in to buy when I bumped into a woman, who stared back at me like she knew me from somewhere.

'Excuse me,' I said, 'but have we met before?'

'Well, the guards wouldn't ask me that, sir,' she said. She looked at my empty basket. 'You must have a small family,' she observed.

Her own trolley contained a week's supply of processed foods, toilet rolls, cans of beer and a gigantic box of crisps.

Later, at the checkout, another woman stared at me.

'Are you the man from Cavan?' she wondered.

So I couldn't resist using the phrase I had heard a few minutes earlier.

'The guards wouldn't ask me that,' says I.

Unfortunately she actually was a guard, off-duty, and just trying to be friendly.

We chatted about the Cavan–Monaghan match while our groceries were being checked out, but it crossed my mind that I had no tax on my car window and so I tried to get away from her when we got to the front door.

'Is that your car?' she asked, pointing at a Skoda Karoq.

'That's amazing,' I said. 'I used to have a Skoda Yeti. But I traded it recently for that Karoq. So how did you know it was mine?' I wondered.

'I saw you getting out of it,' she replied.

'A guard is never off-duty,' I joked, and I was terrified that her car might be parked next to mine. 'Actually, I forgot milk,' I declared, turning on my heel and heading back towards the supermarket.

Not that there was any reason to be afraid of an off-duty guard, but when we were talking football she did admit she was from Monaghan, which didn't help.

But at least in Warsaw nobody spoke English in Carrefour supermarkets. I wouldn't be under pressure to chat, like in Ireland. And so as I planned to head off for Warsaw, I felt I was at the start of a very private journey.

A journey without her. Without anyone. A journey into silence where I wouldn't be bothered by casual encounters in the aisles of a supermarket.

Solitude could no longer be avoided, but could never be discussed. Not with the beloved. Not with anybody.

And we were getting old. The child was reared.

The cats were content. She knew me inside out. And I wondered how she could bear living with me sometimes. There was little I could offer her, and little new to discover with her.

Maybe I should have told her how I was feeling. Maybe I should have joined a golf or bridge club.

Old age is a time for hobbies. People need to fill their days with something. Take up water-colouring. Do the things that they dreamed of doing for a lifetime.

'I've started painting,' I heard an old lady say in the supermarket queue. 'And I've never been happier. I have always wanted to paint.'

But I was wondering why she didn't do it fifty years earlier.

My beloved is an artist. So she lives her own dream. And if I need a bit of leisure I mow the grass.

I remember recently going into Carrick to get petrol for the lawnmower, and I was driving behind an elderly couple in a black Toyota. The woman leaned across the driver's side and gawked out at a fancy house surrounded by roses, laburnum trees and a green lawn.

They drove so slowly that I nearly crashed into their rear end.

Maybe they're grandparents, I thought. Maybe the house they're gawking at belongs to their daughter-in-law, and maybe she's separated, and maybe they drive past her house once a week just to get a glimpse of the children. Or on the other hand maybe they're fascinated by roses.

Who knows how elderly people live out their days or what goes through their minds.

At least me and the beloved had lasted. We had grey hair. We had applied for state pensions. We had free travel, although I didn't like to admit it. And there had been so many changes in Leitrim since we first came. But I didn't admit those either if young people were around for fear they would find me boring.

In the old days there was just one Leitrim – an emotionally impoverished world. A grim island of silence and obedience, of dark fathers with gorilla paws that could clasp a spade like a toothpick and open a ridge of soil in virgin ground with the delicacy of a surgeon slicing his way into living flesh. A world of little shops where the doorbells were cheerless and tinkled with the temerity of a keening woman's cough and behind the counter there was always an elderly lady slicing ham in silence.

And then we came along. The blow-ins. The couples with their babies, and typewriters, and paint brushes, and art materials, transforming little sheds into studios and cottages into homes where you could rear a few children, if you didn't mind the concrete floor in the kitchen and the door of the old Stanley range that never closed properly.

Suddenly there were sculptors from America and England and ceramic artists from Hungary living the dream. The pubs and hotels came alive with hen and stag parties, and the Glens Centre buzzed with radical political theatre and musicians that came from all over the world to gig.

And scattered along the slopes of various hills there were refugees from the urban jungles of Europe, and English boys in cottages or mobile homes who worried about fracking and had lonely hearts, like gardens choked with weed and untended by psychotherapy.

Deeper down in Leitrim's hidden interior there was a kind of Germanic order, a neat organic world sectioned off by high-grade green fencing wire, where people in greenhouses the size of little bungalows nurtured gigantic cabbages and exotic fruits so juicy that John McGahern's father might have self-combusted if he had ever tasted one.

And then came another wave: the Celtic Tigers clinging by their fingernails to the interiors of grand houses; an affluent middle class who were proud of their trim hedges; smooth-shaven men tending their lawns and jawbones with equal attention; shaving in the gym on weeknights and clipping the grass down to the roots on any dry Saturday.

We saw it all, as old people say at weddings when anyone cares to ask them what things were like in the old days.

But I talked less, since I withdrew into myself, and into prayer, lingering in the room of the heart, bowed down in solitude, silenced and emptied. I endured a stone in the mouth, a lump in the throat, a thousand things unsaid. And every unsaid thing was another betrayal that could be avoided by spending even more time alone.

He's at the writing.

He's out in his studio.

He's gone to Warsaw.

The lies mounted up.

The sorrow built like steam in a pressure cooker. Something was about to blow. If it wasn't the heart, what else might have broken?

I needed to get my bearings, not on the outside, but somewhere in the heart. I had lost a compass.

I drove one day beyond Ballinamore and I took a turn to the left, up a small lane, and parked beside the quiet and serene field where John McGahern spent his childhood in the shelter of his mother. I expected to see the remnants of some human habitation, like the track of absent animals.

44 But it was just a field. The house had dissolved, stone by stone, into the air, and only the gateposts stood, with the rusting gate still hanging between them. On the ditches around the sloping field there were alders and hawthorn. The field itself was full of yellow flowers. I leaned on the gate and clung to the serenity of it all for a moment, and Leitrim appeared almost unbearably beautiful, and the sorrow in me seemed like a well with no bottom.

I had seen people struggle with death. They lay for the final few days or hours, holding on, and fighting for life, until some cousin or old friend came from nowhere, and sat at the bed, and in various subtle monologues encouraged them to go. Reassured them that all was well and that the grieving relations would be able to go forward without them.

'Don't be afraid to let go,' the stranger whispers.

It's an ancient message that comes from shamanic voices

hidden even behind the mask of modern culture, but it's a turning point in any dying. After this encounter the person facing death becomes calm and everyone agrees that they have resolved their life.

It's not just that I felt dead inside. There was a lot going on on the outside too.

I went to the doctor and she said I was lacking in vitamin B. So I went on a course to build it up. My muscles were sore in the morning, so I felt like someone had walked over me. There was a continual flashing in the corners of my eyes which I had first noticed a few years earlier, and on that occasion I had gone to an ophthalmologist.

But it had persisted. And now I went again to the ophthalmologist.

We smiled and shook hands, like old friends.

'So,' she said, 'you still have the problem.'

'Yes.'

'It's a mystery,' she said. 'As I said before, it could be a sign that the retina is going to detach from the back wall of the eye, and we have to be vigilant about that. But what's the reason for it? I don't know.'

She squirted drops in my eyes, and targeted the back of my eyeball with a beam of light.

'We'll keep it under observation,' she said when it was over, and she organised another appointment for a few months later.

'Well,' the beloved wanted to know, 'did she find anything?'

'No,' I said. 'Nothing to worry about. It's just old age.'

45

At night I couldn't breathe. I'd wake as if I were drowning, gasping for breath, and the room would feel like there was no oxygen in it.

So all in all on the outside, my body was wrecked. But there was no reason. I had differing symptoms. And I just felt exhausted.

I couldn't walk up the hills that I used to love. I couldn't even walk around the supermarkets without feeling tired.

And I put it down to old age.

'But you're not old,' people would say. 'You're only in your sixties.'

I would smile and say nothing. I felt like I was in my eighties.

Clearly there was something wrong, and since I couldn't put a name on it, I accepted it as a general sign of impending doom, and decided to sort it out on my own, without worrying the beloved. Hence the trip to Warsaw in early 2018 which I booked a few weeks before Christmas.

Seven brass bowls

As Christmas Day approached, the beloved had walked into the room as I lay under the Christmas tree trying to get one of the lights from the tree to shine into the little crib on the floor.

She was carrying seven brass bowls in her hands.

'What are these?' she asked, as she held them up.

'Where did you find them?' I wondered.

'In your study,' she said. 'I was looking for decorations. I thought you had fairy lights in your studio.'

'Those are water bowls I got in India,' I explained.

I had been presented with them by a monk in 1995. For years afterwards I treasured them as precious objects. They were the core of my morning ritual.

I would get up before dawn and go to my studio to meditate. But I would begin by filling the bowls with water, exactly to the brim, and positioning them in a perfect line on a ledge below the Buddha statue. Such a practice is like yoga. It physically focuses the mind. In the symbol of water, I offer my entire world to the gods, the Buddhas, the enlightened mind of being.

They were once so well polished that I could see my reflection on the sides of them as I poured water to the brim. But as the years passed, my practice declined. And the bowls remained full of water and unchanged for weeks. The insides turned green.

They embarrassed me.

I didn't want to see them anymore. Like an ornament that recalls a lost lover, the sight of them wounded me. Eventually I hid them in a white plastic container, in the corner of the studio.

Sometimes I took them out, in a rush of nostalgia, and I would gaze at them for ages, thinking back to the time when I was a student of Rinpoche and would head over to Jampa Ling every second day for meditation sessions, or evening prayers, or weekend teachings. I thought I could rebuild my innocence, my vigour, just like I could re-polish the brass.

But the corroded metal always defeated me and I felt that life had not been an achievement, but just a litany of declines and debilitations.

That winter I'd gotten an urge to clean them. I took them out of the container, and left them on the desk. I went to a local detergent factory and bought five litres of hydrochloric acid. I got an old plastic bucket and soaked the bowls to loosen the oxidised grime.

That worked well.

48

But I didn't finish the job. Like a man who does up an old bicycle in the naive hope that he might begin again; but when he has the job almost complete the bicycle is returned to the shed and gathers grime and dust once more.

So it was with the bowls.

Then she found them in December 2017 and wondered what they were doing on the desk, with a bottle of Brasso and a cleaning rag.

'They are what they are,' I said sadly, and she didn't say anything else, but left them back on the desk. And later that evening I put them in a different drawer, a drawer so dark and remote that they would never come out again.

49

If someone had told me that my arteries were corroded, it wouldn't have pained me more than the corrosion on the bowls, those little brass cups that I had taken home from India and that were the most precious of wishing jewels for me.

By Christmas Eve I had bought a plane ticket online. There was no secret about that. The secret I held from her was the stiffness in my legs; and my flashing eye, which had not improved; and my breathlessness at night; and the fact that I hadn't been walking up any hills recently because I wasn't physically able to.

I talked about buying glasses and writing a book in Warsaw. We discussed the details of my departure in late January. And she offered to drive me to the airport. It would be better than taking a bus, she said. And I agreed, like Judas might have agreed to a sip of wine, or a gesture of kindness from his beloved, at the table of destiny.

I once fantasised about living in Paris and writing in a garret, but it never involved any dark-eyed Parisienne who spoke ten languages and could recite poetry to me as we showered after sex. My garret would have been another solitary room.

Even when I did succeed in getting to France for three months as a writer-in-residence at the Centre Culturel Irlandais in 1998 I spent most of the time going like a yoyo from one beautiful church to another all day long. I was a monk in a medieval world, and I needed nothing else.

That's why I wanted Warsaw again. I needed Warsaw because in old age betrayal is more about turning in on oneself, rather than reaching out.

A couple had arrived to visit us a few days after Christmas, and had stayed overnight. They were both teachers and he had retired but had apparently become a fully qualified therapist. We all ate the leftovers of a turkey, curried into a hot dish and served with brown rice.

By the end of the night the men had separated from the women, who remained in the lounge area, settled on the sofa watching a Christmas movie. Myself and the therapist stayed at the table drinking brandy from Waterford Crystal glasses and talking in hushed voices.

'I am getting very religious,' I confessed.

'You've always been religious,' he joked.

'I'm being pulled back into magical thinking all the time,' I said, trying to make clear that I was concerned.

'Maybe it's age,' he suggested, still finding it amusing.

'I've started praying again,' I confessed.

'What do you mean?'

'Praying.'

'Like what?'

'Like saying, "Jesus Christ, have mercy on me," one hundred times,' I said.

'Fuck me,' he said.

'Correct,' I said. 'Fuck me. Like what's that about?'

'It's nostalgia,' he said. 'Is something worrying you?'

'It's like being lonely all the time,' I said. 'And I feel ashamed of it.'

'Why do you feel ashamed?'

I couldn't answer him.

He poured more brandy.

'Am I having delusions?' I wondered. 'I know there are no angels flying around in the night sky. But I'm talking to them all the time. That's not right, is it?'

We were drunk.

'Going to Warsaw,' I suggested, 'is like going to a desert. Silence is God's language. Am I mad?'

'No,' he said, 'I don't think so. But you might be.'

He was laughing.

'It's not funny,' I said. 'You're the therapist. You should be able to explain it.'

'What are you guys laughing about?' asked a voice from the television lounge. But neither of us was going to answer.

I remember sitting opposite the beloved one night by the fire, before I left, and all my little secrets about physical health and despondency made the silence feel like one more deceit.

It was the first of January. We had spent the previous night watching Jools Holland ringing in the new year, as usual. But this year was different. My flight was booked. I was heading off at the end of the month.

We watched each other in silence. We exhausted every possibility on Netflix. Then we turned off the TV. The fire crackled and the silence thickened until I found it was difficult to breathe.

She looked at me and smiled.

The silence became a wall. There was nothing more I could share.

'You look sad,' she said.

It felt like a kind of grief. As if my silence was a way of saying goodbye. As if I was bidding her farewell at a deeper level. Or else something in me was dying and I didn't understand it.

I was terrified. I knew things were not right. And I would have been happy to crawl into any cradle if there was one close. I wanted to unwind the time, and be again a child with an open heart, and a prayer as pure as a white blossom on the Virgin Mary's blouse.

Certainly I needed glasses. That was one pretext for Warsaw. To write a book and find a pair of glasses. And I wasn't fabricating that.

I had owned many pairs of glasses in my lifetime and I'm always getting new ones. I had never settled on one particular style. I often bought cheap glasses and then I lost them. Or I broke a hinge. Or a little screw fell out. Or the glass fell out and broke. So I discarded them in a drawer and bought another pair.

I went to an optician in Sligo about ten years ago and paid four hundred euros for glasses which I lost a month later on Croagh Patrick as I scrambled to the top. I should have searched for them among the stones, but I was too eager to get to the summit. I reassured myself that I could find them on the way down.

But on the way down I forgot to search for them. In fact I forgot about them altogether, or that I wasn't wearing glasses, until I was in the car park, slipped on a stone, and sprained my ankle.

Some time later I got my eyes tested with a posh optician in Dublin and he gave me an enormous pair of windows. The lenses were so vast, they'd need wipers. And they were heavy on my nose so I ended up with skin abrasions.

After that I became committed to cheap spectacles. One pair after another, until the middle drawer of the oak writing desk in my studio was stuffed with pairs of various shapes and sizes.

Then someone suggested Enniskillen. There was a belief in Leitrim that opticians in the UK would be more professional. In Enniskillen they persuaded me to purchase varifocal lenses. But after a while my nose began to itch.

So if I add up the bill over the years since I first required reading glasses, I might have spent fifteen hundred euros in total. Always the style was the same. Always they irritated my nose. Always I found a way to lose them.

'Did you never notice the amount of opticians there are in Warsaw?' I'd said to the beloved the night before I headed off. 'It's nothing but opticians and chemist shops,' I'd said. 'And considering the price difference, what I save on them would pay for my plane ticket.'

Talking about one thing can be a way of avoiding something else.

The next day she drove me to the airport. We arrived in Dublin just in time for the morning flight to Modlin Airport in Warsaw. I slipped out of the car as lightly as I could. There was no drama.

I went through the boarding gates, walked past the duty free and down to the far end of the building where the Ryanair flights are usually clustered. I watched people queue at gate 112 to board, and I noticed how agitated some of them were. That was unusual; Poles are calm and rational when they queue. And when we got on board people squashed their belongings into overhead compartments and squeezed their big arses into the seats as if it was the last plane out before Armageddon.

I sat in the front row staring at the door of the cockpit, and at the two stewards as they belted themselves in for take-off. They were young Spanish women. I gazed at them in admiration but they didn't see me.

Tiers of a
wedding cake

'OK,' the manager said. 'So let's talk about the top table. How many have you?'

'Well,' the groom replied, 'we have three bridesmaids, and five brothers, and two maids of honour – and then the parents, that's another four.'

'And a priest?'

'Yes.'

'One or two?'

They were not sure about that. The bride had an uncle in Africa. He was a monsignor. He might get home.

'But then again,' the bride said, 'he might not. You know the way it is with Africa.'

On they went, in love, and madly absorbed by every detail, while I sat with a cup holding the dregs of the coffee, and rather than miss a word of their wonderful nuptial joy, or for fear of drawing attention to myself by standing up, I waited till the waitress passed my table so I could get her attention.

'You want lunch,' she declared. 'What will I get you?'

'The beef,' I said.

'I'll bring it down,' she said, and so she did.

The bride stared directly at me just after the waitress left. I thought she noticed me. That her attention had finally gathered me into focus and she might begin to whisper, to become more discreet about her happiness, her anxieties and the notes she had scrawled on the back of an envelope. But she just looked through me, with a blank serenity, like someone in an airport lounge who has left the mundane world and is already on the beach four thousand miles away. She looked at me but she didn't see me.

'What about the centrepieces on the tables?' the manager wanted to know.

'What do you mean?' the bride asked.

'You've got a fish bowl motif,' the manager said. 'That's beautiful.'

'Yes,' the groom replied proudly, 'it's a marine motif.'

'And I need someone to bring the flowers from the church,' the bride added.

'Someone in the family is best for that,' the manager suggested.

'OK.'

'And colours?'

'Pardon?'

'What colours are the bridesmaids?'

'Blue,' he said.

'Royal blue,' she said.

'OK. Well, that's important. Because you need to keep that in mind when you're choosing other colours. You don't want that colour all through the room. So I suppose white for the chair coverings?'

'Ivory,' the groom insisted.

'Like cream,' the bride explained, 'but not white.'

'Well, I can bring you in,' the manager said, 'and you can have a look.'

They intended to pay for a meal for three hundred people.

'That works out at sixty-two euros per person,' the manager said. 'Which is about twenty grand alone for just the dinner. And three servings of wine. How many bottles is that? And the ivory chair covers are extra. But then you'd need a post-drink. You can go with a sparkling wine if you like. For the toast.

'Which brings us to the big question for today,' the manager concluded. 'How many tiers do you want us to cut?'

When we first fell in love we used language to measure each other. To name each other. To lie on the pillow after a climax, smoking cigarettes and asking questions about what our separate lives had been like, before we met. We were trying to explain each self to the other. And as the years went on we grew more together because we shared the same future. The same dreams, hopes, house and a second-hand Nissan. We watched our daughter grow. We planned holidays. We sat at the Christmas table with the same wine glasses, remembering old friends. We laughed together as each Christmas blended with the one before. We flew like birds in harmony, and became so alike that we needed to do less talking.

But we didn't know where the line was between following the harmony of birds, and just going through the motions.

I remember once digging an enormous hole in the garden. We had been married for just a few years. Our love was still fired with the exhilaration of knowing the future was still ahead. My beloved watched from the window, dandling the baby on her hip, and handing me out mugs of tea.

58   Not being experienced with Leitrim soil, I thought that the water which oozed up from beneath the swampy lawn was the sign of a hidden well. I dug like an eejit, until the hole was as big as a First World War trench. Of course it wasn't a well. It was just soggy ground.

But the trickle of water continued, and I became as crazed as the hero in *Manon des Sources*. I had visions of the moment when my shovel would hit the rock and I'd see the clear spring. It would be a metaphor for our new life, a sign that our adventures, risks and desperations as artists were not in vain but rather were being nourished by God, the universe or whatever mythic force of destiny you like to append. The neighbours laughed; they wanted to know why I was digging a grave. And who I intended putting into it.

But eventually the garden took shape. The trees grew. The hole became a pond and turned out to be the centrepiece of the garden. A focal point in an otherwise undisciplined landscape of weeds, shrubs and young trees.

We planted wild irises, which bloomed in July. The trees sucked up the moisture in springtime; but every winter the hole filled with water and mud again.

After twenty-five years the trees reached high into the sky and the land dried out, and the neighbours admitted that we might not be fools after all.

And the pond endured. It became a centre for frogs; they arrived in early March. Each year I would see them wallowing in sexual desire, croaking to their hearts' content while the cat sat motionless on the patio and sometimes moved her paw forward, as if considering a great leap – which caused the frogs to disappear instantly beneath the surface.

I began to envy them, each year as they came like happy teenagers to our hole in the ground where they could enjoy their own kind of Glastonbury Festival for frogs in the mud. And later still the pond became so dry that the frogs went elsewhere. I was left with more memories, and a sense that all good things, even the frogs, belonged to the past. One night in March years after they had gone, I lay awake listening to the water in the radiators, and the noise reminded me of those slimy amphibians, sinking to the bottom of the mud, unloved and repulsive except to each other. And what really kept me awake was remembering all the things we had done since those days, and all the things that were in the past.

59

By the time I finished the roast beef and gravy and the mashed potatoes and green beans in the Abbey Hotel, the wedding couple had lost their mojo. They were still chatting to the manager, but the intensity and excitement had gone from their voices.

The manager was in control, dotting all the final i's.

'Don't forget what we've spoken of,' she said.

'We won't forget,' they promised, exhausted and obedient.

But you will forget, I thought. Eventually you will forget this moment. The tiredness, the boredom, this tedious unpicking through every detail of the day; it will be erased and all you will be left with is the happiness, the loveliness of every perfect thing.

Nearer to me another couple were sitting down. Both of them in their seventies. I guessed they were husband and wife. He was on the phone, making an appointment with a doctor.

He was saying that a thing got stuck in his ear and he needed it to be syringed.

'Yes,' he said, 'ten o'clock would suit me. Tomorrow. Yes. Thank you.'

'I can drive you in,' the woman whispered, before he finished.

'Yes,' he said, 'I have someone to drive me, thank you.'

I put down my knife and fork, wiped my mouth with the serviette and walked across the foyer to the bathroom.

And after washing my hands I decided to wash my glasses as well. The lenses were smudged.

I ran the hot tap on them for a few seconds and after drying my fingers in the Dyson dryer I popped the glasses in for a few seconds. As I came out of the bathroom, the waitress who had taken my photograph, given me a free coffee and then served a wonderful roast beef dinner passed me.

'I like your glasses,' she said.

I felt we were friends at this stage.

'So well you might,' I replied. 'They cost me a lot.'

In fact they'd only cost me a hundred euros, and the truth is that in Warsaw I'd spent very little time looking for them. Perhaps a few minutes here or there, gawking in some optician's window. But I never saw anything suitable. I'd spend hours walking the city streets, noticing nothing but young couples in their twenties, all hooded up and holding hands, or sometimes ogling each other in doorways and pressing their noses together. A delicious grammar of love and generosity swelling their bodies, as they held each other and laughed in the same frosted air that seemed to fill me with remorse as I inhaled one painful breath after another.

Not that we didn't hold each other. But those days were gone. And the cold air of Warsaw was giving me a pain in my chest. As I drank coffee in small cafés admiring the enthusiasm of young people for each other, I tried to accept that even a long-term relationship is a journey into silence and that intimacy, even in a happy marriage, cannot last. Eventually the best of companions need distance. They need space to die.

I noticed churches too, so many of them. More than I had

61

ever noticed before. All around the market square. Near the ice rink in Old Town where plump girls fell on their bums and laughed on the ground. Everywhere, I saw iron doors, and holy men on stone plinths, and I heard bells ringing in the thin air, drawing my attention away from the joy of young lovers and embalming me in a sorrow that I could not explain.

The shiny black bonnet

But we weren't alone in the Abbey Hotel, me and the waitress and the wedding couple with the hotel manager. There was a constant flow of others, in couples or singular, ladies out for a morning coffee after their swim, or young businessmen sorting out stuff on their laptops before some meeting. The man with the sore ear and his wife were gone. But there were old ladies, by the window, talking about their husbands.

I was just back from the bathroom.

'I don't believe he ever got me a present,' one of them said. She wasn't disappointed. 'It was just something he didn't do,' she explained.

The wheelchair was silent in the sunlight beside her.

'One lives in hope,' she joked. 'Oh, but he gave me flowers one time,' she added suddenly, remembering some foggy moment.

'I don't like flowers,' her friend declared.

The waitress wanted to know would I like dessert. She had apple tart or a selection of ice creams. I couldn't choose.

'You could have both,' she suggested.

But before I could agree, a text arrived on my screen from Frank Healy to say the van was ready. So I resisted the apple tart and ice cream, paid the bill and left the building.

I've done it all, Frank's text read. *Lights. Alternator pulley. And a new grille for the front.*

It was going to be either a camper van or a motorhome. That's the one thing I was certain of. But just after the heart attack and during my rehabilitation in the GAA gym doing exercises on treadmills and bicycles, I had not factored in the beloved. It was going to be just me in the van. Because it would keep me healthy. Since I live near Donegal, with all those mountains just waiting for me to find my inner mountain goat, the camper van was going to be the second stage of my rehabilitation course. It would keep me active through the summer. I would park in forests and woodlands, on beaches and cliffs, without being noticed. And though the vehicle was effectively a bed on wheels, or as the General, my old friend from Mullingar said, a hearse for twin coffins, I didn't at first imagine the beloved beside me.

I suppose it's common enough that sometimes the world changes and yet we go on for a short while as if we hadn't noticed.

I spent hours reading ads on DoneDeal, Facebook and Gumtree. I paid a visit to a garage in Dublin that advertised on DoneDeal. But when I got to the showroom they said the motorhome was in a warehouse around the corner. So off I went with a salesman to an old shed in a side street. The salesman opened a rusty lock and unbolted the big corrugated doors and we went inside. He tried a light switch on the wall but it didn't work so we used the torch lights on our smartphones to view inside the banjaxed wreck of a 1993 motorhome. The tyres were flat. The battery in the engine was dead. And the windows inside were crawling with some species of tiny fly.

After that I went to Galway, in February, to look at a big pink Leyland. On the outside it looked like a normal bread van. On the inside it was like a wooden hut, pine panels along the sides and on the roof and floor. There was a basin for washing, and two stove burners. It had been built by a new-age traveller in England thirty years earlier. It was dark and had no windows, but I thought it perfect. I'd be alone in the woods. It was a cave on wheels. I told the guy selling it that I loved it. I could meditate all day long in it. And I made a genuine offer that night, through his DoneDeal account, but he never got back to me.

I kept looking. I imagined myself parked on summer evenings at the ocean's edge. Or by the lakeshore, close to old monastic ruins and holy islands. I imagined walking around lakes and along beaches with aerobic ferocity, and stir-frying vegetables in a wok at the edge of the sand dunes, and washing down fresh fish with a glass of wine before retiring to bed in the back of a dainty van. If only I could find the right one.

I went to a motorhome dealer not far from Lisburn, in the hope of swapping my Skoda for a big white camper with a double bed like Mr Focker in the movie.

The dealer had a vast yard, off the A1, with dozens of white motorhomes lined up in rows and prices displayed on the front windows. And even though I loved my Skoda and its leather seats, I thought it would go a long way as a down payment.

I asked the young salesman if it would be possible to purchase with euros.

'No bother,' he said.

'And would it be OK to trade in a southern-registered car?'

'No bother.'

'And what about importing a camper to Leitrim after Brexit,' I wondered.

'We can do the paperwork,' he said.

But I got a terrible shock when we started talking money. The only thing remotely near my price range was a 07 Citroën Relay van, converted into a two-belt camper, with couches and curtains and low mileage on the clock. It was lovely, but I had no idea it would be so expensive. It was almost thirty thousand euros. So in the end I had to drive away in the Skoda.

And then, just when I had almost given up, I was in Letterkenny one day to do an interview with Highland Radio when a stranger spoke to me in a restaurant near the radio station.

'Are you the man was on the radio this morning?' he asked.

I said I was.

'I heard you were looking to buy a camper van,' he said.

'That's correct,' I replied.

'Well, there's one for sale just down the road,' he said. 'It's on DoneDeal, and it's an old machine but the price might suit you. It just went up on DoneDeal this morning.'

I tried DoneDeal but couldn't find it. So I went home disappointed. But I tried again that night and this time it came up on Google: a Mercedes Vito, 03. It was black on the outside and it certainly looked brand new inside as if it had just recently been refurbished. It had a small sofa seat, a two-ring burner, a portable toilet in the closet. It was perfect.

On the phone the owner said that there was another interested party. Someone had called him the night before but wouldn't give him the full money.

He was looking for 5,500 euros, so I said I'd give him the full amount if I was satisfied after seeing it, but I'd need to be certain that it was available before I travelled back again to Donegal to look at it.

He said I would have first choice if I travelled up.

I drove to Letterkenny the following day, and met the owner, who took me for a spin. Without any hesitation I said I'd take it and an hour later, as we were ironing out the details about the tax book and the insurance cert, the phone rang and the competing bidder offered the full price.

'Ah, but there's a man here who has it taken,' the owner said.

I felt proud of my quick decision. And relieved.

The following morning the van arrived at our house in

Leitrim. It seemed smaller than I remembered, but the interior was in perfect condition, and I was very satisfied. I was imagining myself on the road.

For a few hours I kept going in and out the back door of the house just to admire the shining black bonnet and sleek lines, as the van sat at the gable of my studio.

I got a bucket of hot water, a sponge and washing-up liquid and I cleaned it from back to front. I washed off the soapy water with a few buckets of cold water, and then dried it with a cloth, rubbed T-Cut oil into it and polished it to a bright shine. It felt like bathing a newborn. Or washing a chalice before mass.

I knew it would need a service. It would need tyres. Insurance and tax would be expensive. But by the end of May, it would be ready to go.

Fake beauty

The General once said I only go to Warsaw to get away from the beloved. Which is true enough. But I'd told him that she goes to Warsaw to get away from me.

'You're both trying to get away from each other,' he'd said.

Which I'd insisted was not fair, because, as I'd explained to him, we sometimes go to Warsaw together.

'And did you never hear of Barcelona?' he'd fumed. 'Or Tenerife. Have you no imagination?'

'But we like Warsaw,' I'd protested. 'We're familiar with it.'

However, the last time we talked about going to Poland, the beloved had surprised me by saying we should go somewhere different, and I'd suggested Malaga but she'd meant somewhere different in Warsaw because we usually stayed in Old Town.

We usually got an apartment off the square, and we'd take breakfast on the street, and walk in the parks during the day and then at night, if there was a good old-fashioned Verdi opera at the National Theatre, we'd go and mix with the refined and conservative society of Warsavian opera-lovers.

'If we're going to Warsaw we might as well stick with what we know best,' I'd said. And she'd agreed. And so back we went once again that winter, 2017, to the old part of the city that looks like it survived from the seventeenth century even though it was all assembled from memory, love and old maps after the Second World War.

Old Town has a kind of fake beauty.

The beloved and I lay in bed listening to the sound of vendors in the square and someone playing piano in the apartment below. A Chopin melody slipping up through the floorboards. My beloved asleep on the pillow.

If I was in Warsaw alone I would never go to the opera. I would find it unbearably lonely. And though I would often walk through a park twice or three times a day, I would rarely sit down on a bench, for the same reason as I wouldn't be seen alone in the bar at the opera. I was used to Warsaw with her. But without her, I just kept walking.

Being in Warsaw alone was in itself a kind of betrayal, because the city was what we shared. But at least I didn't book a place in Old Town. That would have been too painful. I would have felt her absence at every corner. Instead I booked an eighth-floor apartment in the modern centre of the city, with a balcony and a view of traffic struggling through sleet, and a glass wall and door between the lounge area and the balcony.

The General had said I was just being nostalgic for an imagined monastic life, for long days of silence in a monk's cell, a silence broken only by the bell calling each monk to the intimacy of the psalms, sung shoulder to shoulder with other monks.

I'd told him that it was not possible to be nostalgic for something unreal. And he'd said that the imagined monastic life was very real. It was part of a man's 'mental arrangements'.

'Every man wishes to be alone,' he'd claimed. 'Not because they ever were, but because they have an inbuilt dream of it. A template wherein they are supreme lord over the universe. That's why you find lions and other animals live alone. But we men live in families and long for that which we can never have: splendid isolation.'

And to be honest I do like to dream about monastic life as it might have been in ancient days, either in the city monasteries of fourth-century Egypt, or on the remote islands off Ireland's west coast. The possibility of what mystics used to call 'union with God' haunts me, the possibility that solitude, once embraced, might deliver up its own special intimacy.

Death can waken old men; it's one last chance to open their eyes in awe. They see it coming and their instinct is to distance themselves from others and be alone so that they can speak to the dark, touch and feel and greet it, rather than allow all that shadow to come behind and frighten them with its sudden presence at their deathbed.

I found myself on the eighth floor of an apartment building not far from Arkadia shopping centre in the winter of 2018, with no one to amuse me apart from the occasional distraction on Facebook, or the often overheard conversations in Costa Coffee. The floors and worktops of the apartment were made of white plastic and there was neither stove nor cat to comfort me. There were no lovely magpies on the balcony either, high above the indifferent city.

A fine May morning

t's a beautiful day out there,' someone said when I was paying for the roast beef dinner.

And before I headed off to collect the camper van from Frank Healy I walked around Roscommon town, going in and out of second-hand clothes shops, coffee shops and the white tents in the town square where the arts and crafts of local designers were on display to the impending June bank holiday.

A radio was blaring out the door of a restaurant, the voice of Joe Finnegan giving stick to various politicians who had won seats on the local council in the recent elections. Further up the street in a newsagent's I heard the voice of Christy Moore singing 'As I Roved Out'. A song I remember from the 1970s when I was a boy in Sligo living in the top flat at 17 The Mall.

There were three young women on the middle floor who played guitars, and an Indian family at ground level who cooked curry in the mornings, which I thought was the most exotic cultural event I had ever encountered.

In the summer me and the girls from the middle floor went to the Ballisodare Folk Festival just outside town, and drank all night. The three girls would make sure to pack guitars into the back of their Renault 4 van, just in case someone might initiate a singing session at the very end of the night, around a campfire.

If that ever happened the guitars were never far away. And they would tune up and play as if having them in the Renault 4 was a fortunate accident. They'd sing their hearts out, dreaming of a life spent performing and an endless road to nowhere with only love and music.

'As I roved out on a fine May morning,' Christy sang. But by this time it was afternoon on the streets of Roscommon, although I was in no hurry to go.

'Who should I spy but my own true lover, as she sat under yon willow tree.'

I loved the way Christy pronounced words. The way he phrased the song. And I loved the song. And I loved my beloved.

In the song the woman is disappointed with the singer because he has been false to her. He has deluded and betrayed her, so she claims. But he denies it. He has been true only to her. Just like I had been true to my beloved.

At the end of the song the singer rues the day he lost her and wishes he was back with her again. That gave me a cold shiver.

A few days earlier Frank had come with another mechanic to our house and picked up the van. Now I needed him again to help me get the van home. So I drove to Ballyfarnon,

74

Frank told me what he had done and I paid the bill and then he drove the van and I followed in the Skoda, as far as home.

Then he hopped into the passenger seat of my car and I drove him back to Ballyfarnon. When I finally returned to the hills above Lough Allen it was 6 p.m. There was plenty of time to prepare for the morning. The lovely black van sat with its nose to the driveway. On the morrow we would head for the hills of Donegal.

We?

And I wondered did I actually say that? We?

And then I thought, Yes. Yes. I did.

The same as before

Warsaw that winter had been just the same as every other time. I had gone back and forth for five years, looking for traces of my great-grandmother in various archives, visiting Auschwitz, and Częstochowa, enjoying the opera in Warsaw or just generally romancing around the streets, the coffee shops and the bars, sometimes with the love of my life and sometimes without her. I'd been a tourist everywhere. I suppose it's the basic condition of modern Europeans.

But this time I went to pray. That marked it out as different. I was afraid, but I didn't know of what.

Everything was the same as before. The same Ryanair flight. The same landing time. The same bus into the city.

Two p.m. on a frozen cold afternoon at the end of January, making my way to yet another Airbnb apartment.

Maybe the woman who welcomed me was a surprise. Or maybe just a distraction. Her name was Lizabeth. Good-looking with denim jeans and a grey blouse. Intense perfume.

'I am the mother of the person who owns this apartment,' she explained.

'And where is your daughter?' I wondered.

'Bermuda,' she said.

'Great.'

'She works in London,' mother explained, with an air of pride. 'She has a degree from Cambridge. But today she is at a wedding in Bermuda.'

'OK.'

I took off my shoes and entered the hallway.

This will only take ten minutes, I thought. And then she will be gone. And I will be alone.

'I have come from Germany this morning,' she announced, in slow, carefully shaped syllables. 'From Berlin,' she added. 'Two hours flight.'

So we had both travelled a long way just so she could give me the keys.

'That's a lot of aeroplane fuel,' I said, joking.

She didn't understand.

'It's a long way to come,' I said, 'with the keys. We all move around so much nowadays, it's amazing that the planes don't bump into each other in the sky.'

She didn't understand 'bump'.

'Crash,' I said.

'Plane crash?' she repeated.

'No.'

'Today?'

'No. The plane didn't crash.'

I would be at home here, I thought, if she would only go. If she would leave me alone. This is going to be my Skellig Rock for a month. I will be living in the clouds. It's perfect. Except for her. I must get her to leave.

Sudden intimacy with a stranger was not in my plan. And yet she was lovely, and pleasant, and she listened to me with intense concentration when I spoke.

Her lower lip was full and sensual. We kept losing each other in conversation. Misunderstanding words. She showed me the dishwasher. And then the washing machine for clothes in the bathroom. And the brushes and stoppers and railings for the shower curtain. She opened a press and showed me where the powders were. The powder for woollens. And the powder for whites. And how to use the railing only to dry small things.

'Small things,' she said.

She was loading me with a lot of detail. And the bathroom was tiny. An hour had passed, and my travel bag was still lying on the white tiles inside the door, and she was still showing me the coffee-maker and the bin under the sink for the rubbish. I didn't know how to get rid of her. But if our little intimacy endured much longer, something new might arise.

Small things.

We'll end up knowing too much. It's too close.

My only issue was the television. And my great regret was that I mentioned it. I asked her how to work it. Where was the remote control?

79

'It's not working,' she said.

She explained that there were two remotes. One for the television set. And one for the satellite box. She plucked them from behind the screen. Held them up for me to look at. But the combination of the two defeated her.

'I live in Germany,' she explained. 'I not live here.'

She stood before the screen, with a remote in each hand, flicking all the various combinations she could manage to think of. And then she asked me did I want to eat.

Viking was a fast-food restaurant that served fish, she explained, and at eight o'clock every evening they reduced their prices by 40 per cent in order to dispose of each day's food before closing.

'We can go and have coffee now,' she said. 'Then you will know where to go every evening if you want fish.'

The restaurant wasn't far away and I thought it would be best to spend the time with her there, drinking coffee, rather than have her linger around the television set any longer.

'Coffee is a good idea,' I agreed.

So off we went, all wrapped up for the cold, in anoraks and scarves. We had the coffee and when I was about to shake hands with her and take the keys, she insisted on returning, so she could fix the television.

It was raining. And dark by now. The lights in the apartments around us were on as we walked. When we returned, Lizabeth stood at the television screen once again, trying to make it work and murmuring something to herself.

She wanted to scream. I could see it in her face. And after another half hour she was exhausted. She sighed. She put down the remotes, like she was dropping two loaded guns, put on her boots and her coats, and was gone without a word.

I could live without television. I could watch Netflix on my laptop. I could listen to nuns on iTunes. I didn't need two hundred East European and Russian television stations to make me happy.

THE REELS

A new pair of togs

The longer two people are together, the more they ask the same questions. Who is my beloved? Where did she come from? And what is her name? And the less they are capable of answering. Marriage is mysterious. Impossible to understand. It is mystical, an ultimate truth which cannot be apprehended by the intellect. In parts of Asia it is called the great koan – a riddle without a solution.

For me the beloved is the one I walk with in the garden at night, when we talk to the trees. She knows their names. And she knows everything about flowers. But in daylight she is practical.

The beloved says things like, 'Those swimming togs are too old. Get yourself a new pair.'

Because the ones I had were too big. They would wrap with ease around Finn McCool's arse, and they flap like a flag around my knuckled knees. But I didn't notice.

It's not that she wants every woman in the Jacuzzi to admire me. But I suppose she doesn't want them laughing at me either. And to be honest, when I see women exit the sauna like a swarm of demented bees as I approach I know there's something wrong. It is the beloved who can name it.

'It's the togs,' she says. 'You definitely need a new pair.'

In the old days women used to chase swarming bees, running behind them with frying pans and potsticks until they dropped. It was considered lucky to make bees drop, and lucky to plant ash trees near the house, and luck was important in lives that otherwise felt as random as flotsam on the ocean. Being superstitious, I have an ash tree outside the window, but my fortune in life was finding the beloved.

The beloved is the one I remember most from all the dinner parties. She was always there, before the visitors came. She was there when they left. I never looked at her, but she was at my shoulder. When everyone was gone we had a final glass of wine and sat in silence.

I remember one particular dinner when they were all there: the young Albanian man who catches pike in Lough Ennell, my friend Fergus who runs a fruit and vegetable store in Mullingar, the woman from China whom we call Little Lotus and the two Russians, mother and daughter from St Petersburg, who have never forgiven me for the time I compared the Irish government to Azerbaijani donkeys. They thought I was insulting the donkeys.

Little Lotus was saying that it's hard to get chicken feet in Ireland. Apparently the claws of Irish hens are exported to China, and chewed, as an accompaniment to beer. I suppose it's all a question of taste. For example, the soup Little Lotus makes from the offal that the butcher throws out is amazing. And her freezer is full of crubeens. And a friend phoned her one night to say that he saw dog meat in Tesco, which surprised him, he said, since Europeans don't eat dogs.

'It was on the shelf,' he said, 'in small tins.' She explained that it was not meat from a dog's body, but rather meat *for* dogs, and she suggested he stop eating it.

There was so much fun and diversity on that occasion that perhaps it could be said that it was the best night of our lives. The company was perfect. In the chronology of time we found a particular moment that was deeper and lighter than ordinary time. We hit a point so deep inside clock-time that it felt like we were living eternity in every second, and that the sun would never set and the moment would live forever.

87

Which it did. Because each one of us still holds it in our hearts. That wonderful night. We remember it for no particular reason. And without many details. But we always say, 'That was the best night.'

And I never thought I'd end my days wrapped up in such kindness: an Albanian, two ladies from Saint Petersburg, a Chinese woman and an Irish grocer. Yet for me, the centre of it all was my beloved. Without her I would not have been there. Without her at the centre, the universe would not be arranged as it is.

When we are young life comes and goes like the ocean tide, and we get washed up in different places and can do nothing about it. But as we get older something in the universe coheres. The friends and family grow around us with the elegance of differing branches on a tree. It's all random and we are powerless in it but when in full bloom the air feels like grace.

Some given thing is received. And this is the attitude that makes for the best parties. Gratitude for being there.

So in any marriage the one who is called beloved is understood as a gift. She is given to me. She makes everything different. Even the camper van.

88   I am occasionally haunted by the epic image of John McGahern's father, who, according to McGahern's memoir, after making his marriage proposal and being reluctantly accepted, headed for Galway and sat on a bench with a bag of oranges, and ate every one of them, alone.

I have eaten many oranges with my beloved. We have gathered many memories. Thirty-four years of small, inconsequential things.

I remember walking on a Donegal beach in the light of the moon with her, when the pub had closed. We walked in silence, and she turned her nose up into the wind, closed her eyes and sniffed the air as if she might foretell the future.

I kept my head down until we got back to the chalet at 2 a.m. We left the lights off and moved about by the moonlight that spilled in the patio door.

When her boots were off I felt a sudden urge to kiss her, but it vanished almost immediately like a tide going out.

Over the years I have come to realise that there is a tide everywhere in the affairs of human beings, and it comes and goes with utter indifference But gratefulness is the key to both the highs and lows.

Sometimes I don't know who the beloved is and then a cloud comes and stretches itself on the top of Sliabh an Iarainn and we both go out to look at it. I glance sideways and see her face and I know her again.

She is the one who came to the hospital on 8 December. She's the one I needed. And not just when the heart failed. There were other times, when colitis, an enlarged prostate or depression landed me in a hospital bed. And it's mundane to say it, I know, but what makes a difference is not religion or faith at that critical moment, but the one who sits by the bedside.

I remember her driving me to the hospital when the prostate was so big that I couldn't pass water, and I pissed in tiny dribbles. I took a bottle with me in the car all the way to Dublin and tried to avoid messing the passenger seat, or being seen by passing traffic, as I squeezed drops of urine one by one into the receptacle.

It was Friday afternoon and I wanted her to leave me at the door and save money on the car park, thinking myself a fearless warrior, but she insisted on carrying my bag to admissions and sitting with me in reception until I was brought to the semi-private room where a blue curtain separated me from another gentleman who was on the same surgeon's list for the following day.

89

I assured her that I loved her, with that heroic quality of a soldier before battle, and she went away down the corridor without looking back. Then the nurses came. And doctors. With questions. Everyone checked my name and date of birth. I suppose if you're going to scoop out the innards of a man's prostate it's important to make sure you have the right man. Though I felt a bit embarrassed repeating endlessly to one nurse after another how hard it was to piss.

The prostate is something men prefer to hide from women, especially those they love; not because they wish to spare the women any particular horror, but simply to spare themselves the shame. But eventually you get used to looking nurses in the eye as you tell them everything.

90

Myself and the other gentleman in the semi-private room spent the evening in dressing gowns, gazing out the window at a chestnut tree, and we were as miserable as if we might be hanged from it. On the morning he was in the toilet when his wife appeared once more, and she spoke to the nurse.

'He's very nervous,' she said. 'He's never been in hospital before. Please take good care of him.'

The nurse assured her that the surgeon was very competent. And then he emerged from the bathroom.

'Hurry up,' the wife said, 'you're delaying the nurse,' and off they went down the corridor, and I was left alone.

But I didn't feel alone. Not even when they wheeled me into the operating theatre, which was a splendid space. I expected a windowless room with searchlights on the ceiling and ether in the air, but in fact there was a huge glass window, and dainty trolleys and young ladies in blue overalls. It was as cheerful as a beauty clinic, and I could see the blue sky over Dublin, although I couldn't ignore the fact that everyone in the room except me was wearing a mask. Someone stuck a needle in my back to freeze my lower body and the surgeon bent low between my legs and dug into me with his microscopic digger, tunnelling all the way up to the bladder through the only available route.

At 6 a.m. the following morning I felt sore. Workers with hard yellow hats gathered outside the window dismantling a Portakabin, and myself and my room-mate, still attached to our beds with catheters, sat up and watched like uneasy rabbits. We speculated that the workmen might be from the bailiff, come to take possession of the hospital, and we joked about the prospect of being evicted onto the street, in dressing gowns, with catheter bags in our hands.

And of course she came to visit. And we joked about the tubes, the bags, the urine and the possibility of future erections.

'It's hard to explain how it feels,' I said.

'I don't really need to know,' she replied.

'Who was she?' my room-mate asked when she was gone.

'That was the beloved,' I said. 'That was her.'

The track bottoms

Some of our friends have lost their partners, and been stranded in grief for years. But we have been lucky. We have shaped each other, like the spiralling sinews of a tree, one around the other. And lucky too because time is a gift that comes dropping slow, second by precious second.

So when I brought home the camper van from the garage, and we both stood in the back yard admiring it, and walked all around it three times, and marvelled at the dainty couch inside, and the closet for a portable loo and the tiny wardrobe, and the cooking stove, the fridge, and even the little television screen hanging from a hinge at the back corner of the vehicle, it was impossible to think of ever turning on the ignition without her beside me.

It was just such fun to share. And it didn't bother me that two days earlier I had envisioned it as simply a method of getting more exercise. Because I know that our moments of joy or sorrow, elation or emptiness, are all accidental and of no consequence compared to the white frost on the mountain or the May bush in the fields, or the clouds over Sliabh an Iarainn.

The wheel of life turns and we play it as we can and everything is true only as far as it goes.

The lesson of marriage is that we contradict ourselves all the time. We change our mind and we cannot hide it.

We say it one way. And the following day we say the opposite. And there is always someone there who knows.

And when the house is empty and all the dinner guests are gone, sometimes I say, 'That was a great night,' and she agrees and we have a last glass of wine, on the sofa, in silence. It's the mystery and magic of marriage; we are together and yet we are miles apart.

Which is why I asked her to come to Donegal with me, the day after the camper van was serviced.

We headed out at noon on the first day of June, although it felt like May because the spring had been slow. We drove up through Manorhamilton and the glens of Leitrim until we got to the main Sligo–Letterkenny road just outside Bundoran. There we headed north, a fast road where Donegal drivers push the pedal to the floor and try to outdo each other with speed, and I hugged the left side of the road and allowed them pass, because the old camper van can only do 80 kilometres per hour at the very best of times.

We stopped at a filling station in Laghey on the south side of Donegal town where the road turns for Pettigo.

The beloved wasn't hungry but I ate a boiled egg sandwich in the van and I noticed an old man sitting at one of the picnic benches beside me.

He wasn't having a picnic. He was just sitting there, waiting. Rotund and still, his eyes were hidden in the fleshy face, like a bodhisattva in contemplation, or like an orangutan bored in a zoo.

When I got out of the van to put my sandwich wrapping into the bin near his table he spoke.

'Not a bad day,' he said.

I agreed.

'You're not from around here.'

I agreed again.

And after measuring each other up for a while in this manner, he told me that he was waiting for a lift and that he and a friend were heading off for a weekend in Mount Melleray.

The hawthorn was still in bloom all around us, its white blossoms dripping off branches in every ditch.

'Will I tell you the best way to see the hawthorn?' he said.

'Please do,' I replied.

'By moonlight,' he said. 'If you get a good moon, you must go into the fields and see for yourself. 'Tis like snow.'

We got to Killybegs by 2 p.m. It was still cloudy, but the wind had died down and the strength of June was growing in the air. Then the clouds moved away and the harbour gleamed beneath a blue sky and there was a bone-dry heat in the day that made us want to lie in the grass and it brought out more and more white blossom on the hawthorn.

'Don't forget your promise,' she said.

'What's that?'

'Every day you must walk more than yesterday.'

'OK,' I agreed, and we walked around the town, up one hill and down another. Because that's what the camper was all about. It wasn't about driving or sightseeing. It was about walking. Walking into new spaces. Landing in open spaces. Parking up, putting on the boots and the leggings and getting out into the fresh air.

'Walking is definitely the best remedy for an ailing heart,' the nurse used to remind us in the rehabilitation classes in Drumshanbo.

'It's like medicine,' she'd said. 'It's even better than a gym or swimming pool.'

I went to the classes every Tuesday for almost three months, lost weight and began to firm up the muscles of my upper body which had been deteriorating for years as I sat at the laptop for hours or just stared out the window.

Myself and a few other crocks in track bottoms, T-shirts and running shoes assembled every Tuesday morning in the Shane McGettigan GAA grounds outside Drumshanbo, named after a young man whose sudden death in New York many years ago was a blow to everyone in his community. We spent fifty minutes there, on rowing, walking, cycling and weight-lifting machines.

I asked the beloved should I join one of the hotel gyms when the rehab course was over.

She just said, 'Make sure you get a proper pair of track bottoms if you do.'

But I was nervous of gyms. Whenever I'm in a leisure centre I often admire young men with magnificent bodies grunting underneath the weight of barbells, but being excessively masculine was never high on my agenda. A vigorous, healthy life of sport and gymnastic exercise doesn't quite turn me on. Donegal seemed like a better option.

And since that moment on 8 December when I felt I might not live until nightfall, I had no inclination to go anywhere alone.

97

We drove non-stop after Killybegs until we came to the cliffs of Malin Beg, beyond Glencolmcille, a rugged bluff of bog and rock jutting out into the Atlantic. It was evening. We parked on the cliff, brushed our teeth, pulled out the bed in the van, spread the duvet, changed into pyjamas and huddled inside after attaching thermal blinds to the inside of the windows, like silver paper hiding us from the world.

In the middle of the night a fierce wind rose up and we grew nervous because the van began rocking like a pram. We decided to sit tight and take our chances, and when the wind died down I got out to piss and stood in the grey light before dawn with the ocean all around me on three sides, and the stillness after the storm felt like someone talking to me.

In the morning we brushed our teeth and drove down by the cliff edge to the village, where we got poached eggs and toast for breakfast in the Oideas Gael restaurant, even though their electricity was out.

We didn't think another windy night on the cliff edge was a good idea. So we drove north for an hour and a half, until we came to the village of Annagry and beyond where the sand dunes stretch for miles between the airport and the beach. We didn't notice a sign saying that parking near the dunes was prohibited.

We were lying in bed once again with masked windows, when we heard a car crawling up the beach. Then the interior of the van lit up as the driver turned his headlamps full onto the van. I squinted out through the slit in the blinds and saw blue lights flashing on the roof of a Garda squad car. We had already knocked back a bottle of wine with two rib-eye steaks that she had cooked on a barbecue tray, which meant neither of us could drive away if we were, indeed, illegally parked. It's not the sort of food I'm encouraged to eat, but if you want to maintain a healthy heart there are moments when love will triumph over all else.

I had visions of being taken to the local Garda station in my pyjamas while the van was impounded.

But the gardaí may have decided we were harmless enough, or else they were just on their midnight break, and wanted to eat their curried chips listening to the sound of the ocean, because after twenty minutes with their lights dimmed they revved up and drove away into the night.

We hugged each other with relief and slept soundly until the dawn woke us and then we walked the beach reflecting on how splendid it was to be alone. Because no one but God could see us in that magnificent wilderness.

And having escaped the guards' scrutiny there was a delicate moment later, when we were on our way south, and I was paying for fuel at a Gala station in Loch an Iúir, and the beloved was buying water. A guard just happened to arrive in the shop for a coffee.

'Good morning, officer,' I said cheerfully as I went out the door.

'Good morning,' he replied. And just when I thought I had escaped, he called after me.

'Come here to me a minute. Is that your van out there?' he asked, pointing at my little black camper. And I confessed that it was.

'It's a grand wee machine,' he said. 'I think I know who owned it.'

He only wanted to chat about the van since it had Donegal registration plates and he knew the previous owner, and not a word about the two old lovers lying in it all night near the beach.

'Let's go back into Annagry,' she said. 'The clouds are clearing. It could be a beautiful day on the beach.'

That's when we passed the Caisleáin Óir hotel and noticed that they had a large car park.

The grey slopes of Earagail reached high behind us and the flat, soft beach of Carrickfinn was somewhere beyond the horizon when we parked on the edge of the little village of Annagry on the west coast. There wasn't a single cloud in the wide-open sky above the van, and a little Aer Lingus plane was slowly floating down out of the blue.

An hour later as we were finishing bowls of soup in the bar of the hotel, I saw the pilot and cabin crew gathering their luggage from the boot of a white taxi, before coming up the steps into the hotel.

'Maybe we should stay here tonight,' she said, 'and park the van in the car park. And spend the day on the beach.'

So we passed an entire afternoon once again on the long white strand, with hardly any other person but ourselves, and in the evening we drove back to the hotel.

By now the hotel was stuffed with young families, and old grannies, unwinding after the tensions and excitements of First Holy Communion services in nearby parishes. Young girls ran around in long white dresses, like little brides, and boys too were in smart suits, though they got less attention. There were grandmothers and grandfathers as well who got fussed over as they negotiated their route in the door with walking sticks or Zimmer frames. There were uncles and cousins home from Glasgow and Manchester. And there were other things to be discussed besides children.

The children were free to run outside and even through the hotel. Up and down the stairs. In and out of the lift. Nobody minded them. Along the corridor to the dining room. Opening and closing the door of the lift. And running all around the huge car park outside, just across the road.

It was a great day of celebration. But it wasn't about the children alone. As with many country weddings, there was a furious sense of community around each table. Cousins, brothers, neighbours all criss-crossed each other, moving from one table to another, and buying rounds of drink. And people were hungry; and the waitresses and waiters rushed in and out with plates of chicken, beef, grilled salmon and pasta. And a long line of men liberated themselves from the nexus of familial ties and stood, each one independently, at the long bar and talked cattle, sheep and weather. They ordered large rounds of beer, lager, whiskey and vodka, keeping their eyes keen on certain tables where their relations sat, with sometimes keen eyes on them.

101

Golden castles

either I nor the beloved were strangers to the coast of Donegal. As a teenager I had learned to touch and kiss in Donegal, on the regular sessions I'd spent in the Gaeltacht every summer at Irish colleges in Annagry, Ranafast and Arranmore. I had spent a winter in Donegal near the airport, overlooking the beach. But the most wonderful moment I ever had along the coastline was in August of 1987, two years after I had met the beloved. She too loved the ancient stones and mountain slopes that skirt the ocean in the northwest. One day we were standing on O'Connell Street in Dublin when we saw McGinley's bus pull in at the Royal Dublin Hotel, and on a whim we decided to throw our bicycles on and head for Letterkenny. From there we got another bus heading towards the coast. And by evening we had arrived at the turn for Magheraroarty just beyond the village of Gortahork. The driver let us off and we took the bicycles and a rucksack with our clothes and rain gear out of the luggage compartment and began a five-day cycle that brought us around the coast,

103

through Bloody Foreland, Derrybeg, Annagry and onwards to Burtonport and Arranmore. We had met in '84, fallen in love and tried to express what that meant and how it might change our lives by going to Italy for a few months in '86. Who knew, but it might have been a turning point, and we might have liked the life out there and never come home.

But in a way the furious excitement of our young love wasn't quite replicated in the sedate heat of modern Italy. It was only in the summer of '87 when we cycled through west Donegal – with the ocean on one side, white with crashing waves against the black cliffs and rocks – that we felt we were living externally and internally in the same moment; living the same mystery of love and attachment both on the inside, in our hearts, and on the outside, in the waves that greeted us at every turn in the road. We were swept into each other's lives and embraced by salty winds each day after another, and secret whisperings of the heart possessed us by night. We had not planned this love. The fact that she was a distinguished artist with an established name in Dublin's little art world, utterly modern in her sensibilities, and me a priest made it an improbable friendship, let alone a love affair. And she had a young son. And I knew nothing of parenting.

It was as unexpected as it was unlikely. People laughed at the comedy of us weaving in and out of traffic in Temple Bar. But it was only on the Atlantic coast that the secrets of each heart seemed to find authentic expression in the rocks and waves along the shoreline.

Despite my heart condition we had steak and mushrooms that evening in the Caisleáin Óir hotel. I was too excited not to celebrate. I was still alive and still with the same person I started out with all those years ago. I asked the barman would it be OK if we slept in our camper van in the car park across from the hotel. He said he'd go and find out.

I looked out the window guessing that the manager would hardly say no. After all, we had ordered a bottle of wine for thirty euros and two dinners. In a few minutes the waiter returned and said there was no problem, so the Spanish Rioja wine arrived and then the slabs of juicy meat and we tucked in like warriors after battle.

We went for a walk later, out the road around the inlet that skirted the sea. We passed a man walking his dog near the beach, which established a strange kind of intimacy, like walking through someone else's dream. We kept walking until long after twilight, as the sun left streaks of light on the western horizon. Then the moon rose high and we could only see the world in blacks and pallid white, but in the end we were surprised by a hawthorn bush so close to the road that we could smell the scented flower that hung in clumps like snow in winter.

When I was a young student in Ranafast all those years ago, there was an old storyteller living there called Seán Bán Mac Grianna. He was a stout little man, and he told a love story as Gaeilge that I learned by heart, so that I could speak every phrase in perfect Donegal Irish.

Bhí teaghlach ina gcónaí i ngleann ceomhar, fadó, it began. (There was a family living in the foggy glen long ago.)

> And they had three daughters and two sons. But as time went on the eldest son went abroad, and the daughters married and there was only the father and the youngest son left at home. And they didn't get on well.

I loved the story. It was simple, mythic and funny. The old man who would come to the Irish college to tell his tales was revered, not just for the number of stories in his own head, but because two of his brothers became writers of published books.

One was Séamus, who wrote a book called *Caisleáin Óir*, about two young lovers who, because of poverty, became separated. They just couldn't afford to marry and the boy was forced to emigrate. But in their youth they held hands, and dreamed that life might turn out beautifully. On perhaps the only beautiful night of their life they sat by the shore not far from where the beloved and I were walking, just across from the hotel, and they looked out to sea.

They were looking out at the clouds gathering beautifully on the horizon.

'*A Shéimí, goidé an cineál tithe iad sin,*' arsa sise, ag amharc ar na néalta, '*atá os cionn luí na gréine?*'

'*Tá,*' arsa Séimí, '*sin caisleáin óir a bhfuil na daoine beaga ina gcónaí iontu.*'

'*What kind of houses are those,*' she says, looking at the clouds, '*above the setting sun?*'

'*Those are golden castles where the fairy people live.*'

It was a charming moment of youthful romance; playfully dreaming of the clouds as some kind of perfect castles filled with wonder and magic. And the metaphor was sustained in the book as the couple resolved to get there. But they never did, because economic necessity and fate stood in their way and their lives were torn apart, and they never saw the fulfilment of that early dream and love.

I'd read the book in the early seventies, when Gabriel Márquez was rising like a giant of South American storytelling, and it had seemed like the simple but mythic narratives of the Mac Grianna brothers were closer to him than to the sophisticated irony of Anglo-Saxon literature which I was studying at the time.

But there was a third brother who mattered to me much more than the other two. And as we returned to the hotel I knew that his grave was just across the road and round the bend in the old cemetery beside the Catholic church. His name was Seosamh Mac Grianna.

I'd read his book too in the early seventies, a strange, dark autobiography entitled *Mo Bhealach Féin* which he completed in the early thirties. Then, in 1935 he slumped into a depressive psychosis, spent years in the solitude of a flat in Clontarf, and when his wife committed suicide in 1959 and his son Fionn drowned in the same year, the writer admitted himself to a psychiatric hospital in Letterkenny, where he remained, alone and as isolated as any despondent monk in the midday sun, for over thirty more years, until his death in 1990.

For me his desire to tell stories, and his mysterious psychosis, made the enigmatic recluse in the Letterkenny psychiatric hospital an enormous shadow for most of my life. I could look at some writers with admiration and others with envy. But for everyone who takes up the trade of storytelling there is always a shadow. Some elder, broken figure who stands like a sentinel outside the writing room, as if it were the darkest hell, and he, just being there, was a warning, not to enter.

I had been a writer, and endured acute episodes of melancholy from time to time, which might be described as depression. But in Warsaw I found in the sanctuary of various churches a shelter from some dark hell that I could only intuit in my gut. I didn't realise how withered one of my arteries was or how close I was to catastrophe.

'You're very quiet,' the beloved said as we got back to the hotel.

'It's just such a beautiful evening,' I replied, pointing back at the inlet, the sand, the distant dunes and the tufts of cloud above the moon. I glanced in the other direction too, as we went in the door, at the Catholic church across the road and the white tombstones huddled around it.

Inside the hotel, we abandoned ourselves to the din of frantic waitering, the roar of a football match on the big screen and the sound of country and western music drowning out the voices of all those families still gathered around the little tables.

I couldn't resist the sense of harmony in the room. The shared understandings, the compromises, agreements, negotiated settlements that made it possible for dozens of mothers, fathers, children and grandparents to be together, and cohesive, in a single space; and yet each face, each expression, contained its own independent gaze, and privacy. It wasn't joy or excitement that pervaded the room, but ease and serenity, a sense that there was a meaning to life and that the meaning was solidly connected to family and community, the delicate balance between individuality and the rightful demands of others.

The beloved held my hand and asked me did I want another drink. I said no. She asked me was I happy. I looked at her and said yes.

'The odd thing is that I can say I've been happy since I had the heart attack,' I confessed.

Spoons from yesterday

A few years ago a woman in Tesco's car park asked me was I happy. She was putting groceries into the back of her navy-blue Almera.

'Are you happy now?' she shouted as I passed, though I didn't even know her.

'Oh, don't mind me,' she added. 'I saw you on television a few weeks ago. You said you crashed, and that you're well again, but I don't believe it for a minute. As far as I'm concerned, when you crash you crash forever. It's like marriage.'

'Are you married?' I wondered.

'Do I look single?' she asked.

She looked overweight, so I said nothing.

'It's the husband ruined me,' she said. 'When we were young it was drink. Then it was Coke. It's always something.'

'Goodness!' I cried. 'Are you saying your husband was addicted to cocaine?'

I imagined a long-haired dropout snorting up the devil's dandruff from a tabletop in some Leitrim kitchen.

'No,' she said, 'it wasn't the drugs. It was the stuff in bottles. He couldn't stop drinking it – that and crisps. Until he was so fat that he got blood pressure and now he's useless, if you know what I mean.'

She slammed the boot shut and got into the car and drove away without looking at me again. It's funny that sometimes one man's story is the story of every man. Sometimes I hear a woman talking of her partner and I feel it's me, or that he is committing my mistakes. It was the husband that ruined me, she had said. And the phrase chilled me to the bone.

112 When I got home I went to the garden and planted a wild rose as an act of contrition. I didn't know for what. I just felt guilty. I stood beneath the big oaks and alders feeling sorry that I had abandoned them, and sorry for the man who ruined his life by drinking Coke, and ashamed for all the times I might have ruined any day for others by carrying too much darkness around the world.

The wind was whispering in the bird boxes, and I was still wondering why a woman would say so much to a stranger in a car park. Apart from the fact that all our sorrows are the same; they are like a single death that creeps into everything and is all-pervasive. It's like a cancer that is all-pervasive in the universe from which every human struggles to be free, and for which every human feels the same guilt.

I remember many years ago sitting in the kitchen, on a Sunday morning, with a boiling kettle. The chicken was in the electric oven. The range was only just lit. Two firelighters blazed beneath six briquettes in the firebox behind the door. Outside it ought to have been summer but it was not. The clouds were grey and the wind blew from the north and the rosebuds and the willow leaves were scattered on the roadside.

I was missing the comfort of mass, the Sunday-morning ritual I had grown accustomed to.

As a priest I got a sense of belonging every week when people gathered around the altar. Even when I retired from my ministry as a priest in 1985 I still said an occasional mass in the old folks' home in Cavan where my father had died. But eventually I knew that I needed to give up that ritual, if I was to go forward in a new life. So the last mass I celebrated as a priest was intentional and sad, in July of 1986. I spoke the words, and read the prayers for one last time in the quiet oratory of the nursing home on the tenth anniversary of my father's death. I spoke all the words with the same reverence and hope as I had done at the beginning. And I wondered why I was leaving.

How would I survive without the comfort of ritual?

Where would I find another sacred space? And how could I ever be happy if the notion of sacred space was, as the modern world implied, a complete cod?

For a year or two afterwards I experienced a low-grade choking in the throat whenever I cycled past the doors of city churches as weddings or other festive events were being celebrated and men in morning suits or brides in white gowns waited outside the doors for the ceremony to commence.

113

The beloved endured it as one does with a partner who has recently been bereaved. I tossed and turned a lot at night as if I was wrestling with a ghost. I drank a lot and dragged hangovers around on my back like a sack of coal.

I felt poor, and undernourished in my heart. One Sunday morning in Ranelagh a bride in a silk gown emerged into the sunlight from the Church of the Holy Name, on Beechwood Avenue, her fresh husband beside her with sparkling white teeth. Everybody was happy and full of grace and drenched with confetti. Except me. I had locked myself out of all that joy.

And for consolation, I often listened to the mass on the radio on Sundays, comforted by that quaint fragrance of the past.

'We welcome those listening in hospital or sick at home,' the radio priest declared with solemnity each Sunday, and I felt secretly included.

One morning we'd been lying in bed when the newscaster on RTÉ had announced that Bishop Eamonn Casey had been accused of fathering a child by the child's mother. I'd leaped up in the bed with astonishment, because Casey had been the chairperson of a committee I was on when I had been a cleric – an advisory committee on youth affairs. We met in the bishop's residence in Galway a few times a year on Sunday afternoons. He would conduct the meeting between three sofas in a grand drawing room of the palace, with coffee and buns served by a woman who came and went

114

without introductions. The bishop behaved extravagantly, his thoughts were always off the cuff, he was consistently over-excited and he smoked huge cigars. Brandy would be introduced at the end of the meeting, lavish dollops in cut glasses. By the time we got to the dinner, served in another room, with the bishop at the head of the table, we were well-oiled, and the bishop rattled out one anecdote after another about how he had championed this or that cause against various adversaries: the social services in London, the county council in Kerry, the other bishops on the hierarchy, or even the Irish government in his advocacy of Third World issues when he was director of Trócaire.

115

By the time the taxi came to convey us to a nearby bed and breakfast most of us were generously inebriated, although the ones who always made me uneasy were two young tailor-suited clerics who avoided the alcohol and conducted themselves with the impeccable discretion of men with careers.

I got a hand-written Christmas card from the bishop every year. He signed it himself. Eamonn. It felt sincere.

But when I abandoned my position in the clergy, the Christmas cards were terminated. What I had taken to be personal was in fact a hollow protocol, swiftly dropped when I dissented from the official church.

I hopped up in bed because to hear of his disgrace seemed like a straw in the wind. He had been a hero of the institutional church, perceived to be an enormous character of integrity. If he could be shaken, then the entire edifice was liable to crumble.

And his leaving was not without irony.

A few days later a black Mercedes whisked him to the steps of a waiting plane. His exit from public life resembled nothing more than the style of many cowardly dictators who had fled in similar fashion from the countries they had destroyed, and who would have been robustly reviled by the same bishop.

And the years that followed only proved that Casey's cowardice was in the halfpenny place compared to the full rot within the celibate church.

The discrediting of clerics worldwide, and the corruption in the Vatican, was demonstrated so forcefully by one documentary after another, by accounts of lives destroyed, of suicides, duplicitous bishops and depravities theretofore unimagined behind the clerical curtains, that it all prevented me from feeling any further ounce of nostalgia for the world I had escaped.

And if I missed the vestments and the bells and incense and the ritual just a little bit, then I was happily compensated when I walked in the door of Jampa Ling Tibetan Buddhist Centre in west Cavan in 1995. I could say with honesty that I had let go of Christian practice, and in its stead I had turned towards Tibet, where they had just as many bells and chimes and incense sticks as the pope.

When I first took refuge in the Panchen Ötrul Rinpoche, and prostrated my full length before him, and declared my faith in the four noble truths of Buddhism and in his worthy authority as a teacher and lineage holder, connecting him directly back through Tsongkhapa of the fourteenth century in Tibet to the Buddha Shakyamuni in India, hundreds of years before the birth of Christ, I did so only after I had shared one important fact with him.

'I was ordained a priest,' I said, 'and I have not renounced it.'

He laughed. 'Very good.'

I was grateful for his acceptance. And in that context I became his student.

He became my refuge, and I shared long silences with him, and when I sat on Sunday mornings by the range I had no further sorrow or remorse for the life of Christian things or thoughts or images. They were part of the past. In the early days I set aside a box to house my old prayerbooks, chalice and golden paten that was once used to hold the bread at mass. They were nothing more than artefacts from a bygone era. The rituals of Christian faith had been washed out of me over the course of a decade by the gradual discrediting of the church, by their refusal to follow through on the promises of social justice that had been made in the documents of the Vatican Council, and by my new-found faith in the wisdom and riches of Tibetan philosophy that became available to me through the holy monk in Jampa Ling.

From then on, every Sunday morning, when the child was young, I just sat in the kitchen with the beloved as the

117

potatoes boiled and the chicken roasted away in the oven. I sat quietly and lit the fires.

Sometimes she'd wash the child's hair. And I'd sit at the range, without any radio to interrupt the sound of her voice in the bathroom, talking shampoo, towels and horses with her daughter.

I felt blessed by the universe, which was the word I began to use as a substitute for the word God. And I realised that life was endlessly comic.

118

The angel and the fish

When I was a child I was happy. Perhaps because I prayed. I knelt at the bedside every night and whispered little mantras in the dark.

There are four corners on my bed.
There are four angels around my head.
Matthew, Mark, Luke and John.
God bless the bed that I lie on.

It was safe, then, to dive onto a soft mattress, dressed in sheets and pillowcases. And sixty years later, after all my coming and going with God and religion, I'm not much different.

The four angels – Matthew, Mark, Luke and John – were boys with feathered wings in my imagination, and they became my imaginary friends. They were soft like fog or watercolours, rather than substantial. They travelled around in my imagination when I was in primary school. They sheltered behind my eyes. They whispered in my ears. They even flitted about in the corner of the playground. I would leave my schoolmates at a distance and loiter in a corner, beside the wall where I could talk to these phantoms.

When I became a teenager the four willowy angel boys, who had been so like a soft pink mist or cloud around me, became more substantial; Matthew, Mark, Luke and John mutated into John, Paul, George and Ringo, collectively known as The Beatles. They turned into substantial gods.

I saw them on television, and knew them instantly. On Wednesday afternoons, when the school closed for the half day, and all my classmates were sucking Coca-Cola through straws in the Central Café down on Bridge Street, I retired to the dark dining room of our stuffy middle-class suburban semi-detached and turned on my father's black box gramophone and slipped on a long-playing record called *Rubber Soul*, which I was convinced was the best album The Beatles had ever recorded, and I would sing for an hour or two, in harmony with my four wonderful friends.

I forgot about angels, and I stopped saying prayers at bedtime, and like other children I began wrestling with sexual desires at night.

One summer when I was eleven I had experienced a sudden awakening in the Gaeltacht, in the front room of a bungalow, on a bunk bed with a boy my own age. It was a long, slow kiss between children. And after an hour of him, he held me knowingly. We embraced in a beautiful dry shimmering which changed me. His kisses felt like the touch of a strange and beautiful other; it was as close to what adults called God as I could imagine. And when the ecstasy was over, the world seemed drab and mediocre, but I knew that it was also peppered with moments of intense and beautiful self-forgetting.

I had fallen in love. And when I came home from that holiday I turned my attention to the even more amazing possibilities of finding intimacy with girls in the dancehalls of Cavan and Longford and the carnivals at Lavey Strand and Drumlish on summer nights. And perhaps I have never fallen out of love since. There's always someone, a person, cat or ghost that touches me. Because love is a capacity.

The wonder of it lies in self-forgetting, that same abandonment that was once required to dive off the top of a tar barrel into the waters of Annagh Lake near Butlersbridge when I was ten years of age.

After my first erotic encounter in the Donegal Gaeltacht, I surrendered to poetry, sunsets, invisible deities, even ritual and prayer, and the transcendence of Loreto girls on their bicycles. I surrendered to girls everywhere, and to fish in the waters of Lough Oughter, with a sense not of shuddering, but being shuddered. A sense not of taking anything from the other, but of being taken.

I had no choice. They came as they willed, gods and heroes, angels and fish, and creatures of erotic perfection, by night or day. I prayed and fell in love with equal devotion. Nobody told me that an erotic life was incompatible with prayer. I got it mixed up in the sense that I thought erotic life was prayer. When I wasn't being tossed at night in furious embraces with phantom girls in school uniforms, I went with ease into the arms of any ghost or saint that might have me, and to the comfort of angels and the Mother of Jesus.

Walking the streets of Warsaw at sixty-four years of age, alone for an entire month in winter, hadn't seemed like the fulfilment of that young spirit. It had felt like the opposite, like everything I had been and hoped for was dead. And I'd walked so much during the first week there that my left leg had gone numb right down the thigh. It had worried me, so I'd asked my friend Doctor Google what it could mean.

'Cause of numb leg,' I'd typed in the search space, and I'd got half a million options.

According to Doctor Google, tight underpants might cause severe numbness in the leg. So clearly I had found the problem.

I went out and bought an enormous pair of trousers, waist size 45, and an XX Large underpants, although when I returned to the apartment and tried on the new clothes for an hour or two my leg was even worse.

I lay on the bed for two days to rest it until the numbness began to thaw and sensation returned.

I ventured out again, though it was minus 2 on the streets and sleet was sweeping across the parks and pavements, leaving a white sheen on the world like scattered salt. My trousers were so loose that my underpants fell down, inside the trousers. I bought a tin of tomato soup at a nearby shop, returned, undressed and felt the leg. It was still numb and so I faced another day or two indoors.

I opened my Kindle and downloaded the Philokalia, a complete compendium of writings from the early Desert Fathers. I had heard that Evagrius, a monk of the fourth century, was worth studying on the subject of despondency, and in desperation I began to trust old monks and ancient mystics, and a multitude of Orthodox Christian websites, rather than Google, despite their flowery language and propensity to blame all ailments on demons rather than scientific or medical diagnosis.

123

Every so often I would come across some tall bearded young man with an American accent on You Tube, wearing the robes of an Orthodox priest, swaggering around the microphone and smiling with the understated steel of a four-star general as he spoke about the evils of the modern world. But I found that if I closed him off before I heard whatever guff came out of his mouth, he didn't bother me, or disturb the benign feeling that was growing in my heart for the wisdom of the ancient Christian tradition.

Those solitary explorers of the inner mind, who lived in the deserts and in caves or on wild cliff-edge monasteries on the west coast of Ireland, before modern psychiatry was invented, spoke in a poetic language that drew me in, phrase by phrase and word by word.

Five nuns

A kiss had a beautiful significance in the flowery language of that ancient religion. A kiss was not just a kiss; it could be a metaphor.

The entire world was described by ancient mystics as a kiss. It was where the invisible world touched this world. A kiss was nothing in itself. It was what two people did, and it was how they connected.

Similarly, the earth itself was not substantial; it was more like a veil, and the point at which the ancient monk engaged with it could be described as the kiss.

It was a point of exquisitely beautiful connection between the little monk there in the desert who viewed it, and the mysterious other beyond the veil who in the eternity of that moment was touching the surface of things as intimately as a lover.

Florid ideas, but in the face of a numb leg they calmed me.

And when the leg had improved, those ideas had kept me going for hours, as I wandered aimlessly around Warsaw without knowing where I was heading, but that I was in the slipstream of my own devotional fervour – a kind of heat in the heart that kept me walking.

At the junction of every new street I wondered where I might end up. I felt I was not unlike a seventh-century monk who might sit in a boat with his oars up and wait for the tide to take him where the tide wished.

One day I bumped into five nuns, huddled together on a street outside a restaurant. I gawked at them because even in Warsaw, a city of strong religious orthodoxies and well-regulated religious life, nuns have become as scarce as hens' teeth, and are not as often seen in public as they were in the old days. Whenever I did notice one, flapping in her black robes or gleaming like a beacon on a street corner with a white veil, I tended to follow behind them out of curiosity, and I suppose an unconscious yearning to belong in their world of gentle certainty.

They were huddled in a circle. Three of them were elderly but sprightly and thin, like nuns are supposed to be, and the other two were young and plump. The older ones were in black from their covered heads to their sandalled toes. One of the young ones had a long black habit but she wore no veil, and I guessed she might be a novice. Her cheeks were flushed and she bubbled with rustic cheerfulness. But the other young nun, also in a long back robe, wore a white veil and had a guitar case strapped on her back and her face tilted to one side like she was yearning for something.

I couldn't stop wondering what might be in her heart. Perhaps she dreamed of being in a folk group. Perhaps she was lonely. Perhaps the guitar and the quiet longing in her eyes revealed some disappointment with life.

Maybe she was in despair and didn't actually believe in Christ or any god at all. Maybe she regretted all the human intimacy she had abandoned the day she robed herself in black.

If that were the case, then her struggle was no more tragic than mine. Because deep down, all my relationships with the saints in Egyptian deserts, the angels in heaven and even Christ himself who stood just beyond my fingertips when I surfed on Orthodox websites didn't imply any religious convictions in the traditional sense. I knew from having to survive alone with a sore leg that believing in any magic is beneficial if it gets a person through the day. Faith for me was always a survival mechanism. And besides, most spiritual paths conclude in disappointment, if not sorrow.

Maybe the young nun should try Buddhism, I'd thought. It's not so much a religion as a psychotherapy, and it doesn't disappoint as much as Christianity, because it doesn't offer as much. The truth is that I'd sell Buddhism to the cats if I could. In fact I tried once, at home, when I was idle and had nobody to talk to only my little furry companion.

When the beloved was away, and the sleet was falling on the roof and the little pot-bellied stove was crackling with logs and the cat was curled up on the sofa staring at me like a grumpy monk, we would fall into a deep and fantastical relationship.

I want chicken, the cat declared.

'You're not getting chicken,' I replied.

127

But your beloved gives me chicken, the cat protested.

So I corrected him. 'She gives you the skin of the chicken.'

He rolled on his side, turned his backside and the remnants of his testicles towards my face, and stared at the flames in the stove.

'She gives you scraps when she has roasted a chicken,' I continued. 'But I don't roast chickens. I live out of plastic bags and cartons. I give you dry food. I don't make a fuss about you like she does. She favours you in particular, as opposed to all the other mangey cats in Leitrim. She differentiates. She sees you as special. But I don't consider that very Buddhist.'

She's kind, the cat muttered. *That's Buddhist.*

'But she's killing you with kindness,' I replied. 'Then she goes away and all you have is me, and a bag of dried nuggets. And you won't eat them, because you're spoiled. How could you ever survive in the wilderness if you don't take what you get.'

I don't live in the wilderness, he whinged, his eyes watering. *I live with you. I thought you liked me.*

'I refuse to make a fuss about you. I'm trying to be emotionally detached,' I shouted, and I was very nearly getting the broom from the kitchen.

You call yourself detached? the cat replied, *but you're as cross as a bag of cats.*

Admittedly I was a bit irritated.

Are you annoyed with me? he wondered.

'Yes,' I said, 'I'm thoroughly frustrated with the way you're looking for a chicken that I don't have.'

128

You do have chicken, the cat screamed. *I saw little bits of chicken last night, floating in the Thai soup you took home from the takeaway.*

I saw him bang his paws on the floor and tears came out of his eyes, and I thought he looked remarkably like Michael Gove.

You do *have chicken,* he insisted.

'OK. OK. So I have chicken.'

I went to the bin in the kitchen and took out the white plastic container from the Chinese takeaway, hoping to find the dregs of the soup, but not a single scrap remained.

Then a new idea arose in the universe. I took a chicken stock cube from the pantry, warmed it in a saucepan with a few spoons of water, and poured it over the dry food.

'Come out here and see what I've got,' I shouted from the pantry, because he was still stretched at the stove.

I waved the bowl of nuggets and warm chicken stock under his whiskers. His nose twitched.

He sniffed the bowl for a long while. Walked away. Then returned.

Finally he looked at me and uttered a barely audible sigh, as if to say thank you. And he started munching. Munching and devouring, and halfway through he looked up at me again and I felt ashamed that I had been angry with him.

When he was finished we both sat at the pot-bellied stove and I put on another log, and the sleet was still falling outside, but we were cosy enough. I was looking forward to his company for the rest of the evening.

Perhaps I was a cat, I thought, and am now reincarnated as a human. Or perhaps he was a human and is now reincarnated as a cat. Who knows?

I was missing my beloved, and so I had taken my frustration out on him. But some rhythm in the universe brought us together, like two monks in a monastery.

He was missing my beloved's cooking, so he pestered me. But with compassion and the imaginative power of a human brain we had found a solution: chicken stock cubes. Now we could both sit happily at the stove for the rest of the evening. Free from loneliness. Detached from further desires, in a calm and shared state of contemplation.

But then he surprised me again by heading for the back door.

'Where are you going now?' I wondered.

Out for a shite, he said.

'I thought we were going to practise our Buddhism together?' I protested. 'I can do my Tara practice and you can do mouse practice or whatever you imagine as beautiful floating in front of your face.'

He didn't even reply. He walked into the back yard and dissolved in darkness, as if he had achieved a level of supreme detachment far beyond my comprehension.

By now the nuns had agreed among themselves what they were doing and they began to stride the broad pavement down Nowy Świat in a row of five, as people dodged them with the respect due to nuns.

I walked behind them. I wanted to tell them it's not possible anymore to live as they are living. In the end they will fall back on their own self, no matter what cloister they hide in, and failure will become part of their bone marrow as the pages of their prayerbooks turn yellow and age wrinkles their hidden faces.

I followed them in their hollow cheerfulness, my eyes on the young one with her sad guitar strapped to her back, as they all went into the Church of the Holy Cross.

I too blessed myself at the door and went deep inside, and there they sat, up in the front pew, whispering some prayers or psalms in Polish. I sat in the back pew and felt less isolated than I was outside. Because even this remote contact with the hem of their garments comforted me.

I sat for half an hour, until my leg thawed. I was warm again. And then the nuns withdrew.

They gathered up their emotions, wrapped their long black robes around them, zipped up their shining black anoraks and genuflected with slow attention to the red sanctuary lamp hanging above the altar.

The Church of the Holy Cross is like the heart of Warsaw. The heart of Poland. It's the church that the Germans blew up after the Warsaw Uprising, a heroic moment in the summer of 1944 when the Polish underground resistance led by the Home Army tried to liberate Warsaw from German occupation.

A bronze statue of Christ stands outside the main door. It had ended up in the rubble when the Germans were finished, but in the fifties the building was restored, and Christ returned to an upright position.

'Lift up your hearts,' he said.

Even Chopin's heart is here, embedded in a pillar in the main hall of the church. Although the nuns didn't stop to notice that, as they headed for the back door, refreshed by their prayers and as confident as magpies.

Which is not to say that I dislike either magpies or nuns. But of the two it's certainly less easy to love the magpies. They are unlucky. Or at least some people say so. Their black and white feathers become a metaphor for tragedy.

In Leitrim we had a dog who lived outside in the yard, and was given a bowl of cereal every day. One morning I was woken by the sound of battling magpies gorging on the leavings of his dinner.

Before the magpies came there were goldfinches, coal tits, thrushes and blackbirds. But the dog's dinner changed the ecological balance.

And it's even stranger how the tiniest fracture in the best relationship, like failing to agree about how to empty the dishwasher, can grow into a monstrous resentment, and an unfortunate magpie might just sit on the clothesline at the wrong moment and be forever seen as a harbinger of sorrow. As a signal of how much unquiet is hidden underneath the surface of things.

I withdrew from the church despondent, and did not bother to genuflect. I wrapped up in the porch, stared at a beggar woman who had been sitting on the wet ground just outside, as if she were an enemy, and began to trek back to my apartment.

I had lost interest in the five nuns, and hobbled home on a limp leg. I opened up the laptop and flipped through the pages of my Facebook friends.

Seven minutes earlier Natasha had posted a picture of an icon. Natasha was a Russian who worked in the theatre in London. I had met her through an actor friend who had been in the musical *War Horse*, which I went to see when it first opened. Natasha was with him at the bar – a dark-haired woman in a black lace dress with passionate views about theatrical design, Vladimir Putin and wild horses. She loved all three with equal intensity.

We got on well and met on a few other occasions for coffees whenever I was in London to see stage plays. She had a daughter married to an Irishman and eventually we became friendly enough for her to invite me to a dinner in her apartment just after Christmas one year. The beloved was with me, and Natasha's daughter and her Irish husband were also at the table. It was a wonderful family celebration in early January.

The icon Natasha posted on Facebook when I was in Warsaw depicted Jesus on the Cross, and though it was dark and ornate it was also dramatically different from the twisted Jesus writhing in pain that I had been accustomed to in western churches. In Natasha's icon Jesus was not in agony.

Far from it. He looked serene, with his arms outstretched, rather than nailed to the wood.

It must be the beginning of Lent, I thought, in the Orthodox Church, and suddenly I loved her for posting her icon.

'My grandfather was a priest,' Natasha had said to me, at that Christmas dinner, when myself and the beloved visited.

The dining room walls were white, and the curtains were white, and the Christmas tree was white, and there were blue lights on the tree.

I said, 'Pushkin was shot in the snow.'

She said, 'Would you like to go to Saint Petersburg?'

I said, 'I'd love to; I think Russian writers are very spiritual.'

Then she poured me another vodka. I was looking at the icons in the corner of the room.

'We Irish have lost our sense of the sacred,' I concluded. 'We need Russians to invigorate us again.'

'You are correct,' she agreed, as she refreshed my glass yet again.

'In Saint Petersburg,' she said, 'we believed in Father Frost, and he was invisible, although he came on Christmas night, with his granddaughter, and they always dressed in blue.'

Stuffed sea bass, Russian salads and herrings wrapped in potato, onion and beetroot were spread on the table, as she poured more drink.

I thought she said, 'This is called heron-in-a-fur-coat,' as she pointed at one dish.

'What a wonderful image!' I declared. 'A heron in a fur coat!'

'No,' she said, 'not heron! Herring! It is called herring-in-a-fur-coat.'

'Well, it is delicious,' I said.

'So now we will have goose for main course,' she declared. And so we did. But we didn't have music, which was a pity – just more vodka.

I told her that I always liked music with dinner.

'Ah,' she said, 'now you sound like Tolstoy.'

After the meal she opened another bottle. Her daughter and partner were still at the table, as was the beloved, but I moved to the couch. Natasha was tidying away the dishes. The beloved was asking the young man what part of Galway he was from. I was absorbed with the little icon corner; the red lamp beneath an icon of the nativity that had been burning all through our meal time.

Hi, Natasha. I'm in Warsaw with a sore leg. And it's very cold outside. How is the weather in London? Happy Lent.

I put a 'Like' beside the icon of Christ and posted my message.

And then I opened Google Maps to see if could I find an Orthodox church in Warsaw.

The remembrance reel

One escape from Christ on the streets of Warsaw was to play with alternative mythologies.
Through my years of familiarity with Tibetan religion I was able to construct an image of Buddha sometimes,
and from that image I reconstructed everything around me.
As if my immediate environment, the bit of Warsaw that
penetrated me, did not exist of itself, but was instead an expression of a loving Buddha being.

I especially liked Tara, the female Buddha, a mother figure
in Tibet as pervasive as the Mother of God in Europe.

In Tibetan iconography Tara is sixteen and her body is
white and crystal clear. She sits in the lotus position. Her hair
is black and adorns the top of her head in a crown pinnacle
flowing down her back. And she wears a jewelled crown.

And out of her I imagined all the world around me. As if
everything was the surface of her being. I walked through
an emanation of her compassion. I treated all phenomena
around me as if they were fragments of a dream, and Tara,

Compassionate Ground of All Being, was the well from which they sprung.

Like any visualisation used in therapy, in grief counselling, in healing rituals or meditations, it was only a mental trick. But it worked. It was like putting on a soft light in a room that imbues the space with a warm glow; so my mental agility allowed me to see the things around me as if they were glowing with the vibrancy of love.

When I was walking in the freezing fog I sometimes took this Buddha with me.

138   It was a daft way to promenade the city; but most people on the street had smartphones and were inhabiting their own cosmologies and virtual realities all the time. Even listening to the news, or podcasts through earphones, is the creation of another hidden cosmology. And who is to say how many people walking on the pavement at any moment are not possessed by demons of desire, anger or rage, as they chatter into microphones, barely conscious of where they are walking in that present moment.

Everybody lives in wonderlands of virtual delight, of heroes and demons, and it could be said that nothing much has changed from medieval times to the present day except that our dreams and fantasies have been incarnated as material objects or addictive narratives in the universe of screens. That's how I justified my Tara practice.

But my pilgrimages to churches, every morning, were a different kettle of fish. I argued with myself that they were merely acts of remembrance. But they were more than nostalgia. The Christian faith was taking hold of me again, and it felt like a betrayal of the beloved each time I crossed the door of a another church. I was being drawn into a kind of exclusive solitude. And the shadow of Christian institutional antagonism towards women only heightened the sense of betrayal.

The beloved knew I was struggling with the work, but I was thousands of miles away and there's only so much can be shared on a phone line or a Skype connection.

Some days I just felt like I couldn't go on much longer, feeling as exhausted as I did. And on those days I didn't phone anybody.

139

I felt so tired of writing that perhaps I hoped this time in Warsaw would mark the end of the books, and the end of writing.

Perhaps I had done enough.

Like Mac Grianna long ago, I had now come to the point where the well had dried up.

And to an extent it had. By the time I returned from Warsaw I was convinced I would never write another book, and I even stopped writing columns for the newspaper. It was the longest and most barren period I had ever experienced as a writer and it only ended when they gave me a stent and the blood in my veins began to flow normally again. Only then did I return to writing columns and the words began to flow from my heart onto the pages of this book like water from a new well.

So there was no danger of me ending up in a psychiatric hospital for decades, like Mac Grianna, but for that year my future felt extremely bleak.

I went to the doctor regularly. I had no major issues either with my sugar levels, cholestrol or blood pressure. But despite there being no signs, physical or emotional, that anyone could pick up on, I was ill. My heart was under pressure. My body was deteriorating.

Especially in the freezing fogs of Warsaw that winter. If it wasn't an arse, it was an elbow. Legs went numb. Muscles turned into fatty flab. Flashing continued in the corner of both eyes. Blurred vision was as common as little faint pains in the chest. Headaches. A sore neck. A very odd pain in the left arm. A general inability to do much apart from walk for a few hours and then collapse for the evening in the apartment, hugging Facebook, and trying to convince myself that it might be the cold weather that was affecting me.

But that didn't explain why I woke at night, struggling for breath as if I were drowning.

And eventually even religion let me down. I woke one morning after about three weeks and felt like a stranger in another person's flat. I opened up my phone and gazed at my laptop as if both of them might belong to someone else. I imagined them as orphans, just as personal items become orphaned when somebody dies suddenly and all their bits and pieces lie strewn about their desk, and on their bedside locker.

I felt intensely mortal, and no amount of clinging to religion can comfort a dying animal.

To put it in the florid language of medieval times, God had abandoned me abruptly. I was tired of traipsing around churches, and moaning to myself like a dying cat.

So I shifted my focus to secular things. To concerts and art galleries and operas, to move the heart.

If death is a bitter and sour ending that signifies nothing, then let's get on with it, I thought.

I avoided nuns. I stopped noticing them. I didn't hear any more bells. And I began reading Beckett, on my Kindle.

I looked again for glasses. Humouring myself by saying that at least I would look well in a coffin. And I tried to tune in to the modern world whenever I was in a coffee shop.

A few days later in Starbucks on Nowy Świat I'd been drinking a latte with an extra shot, sitting with my back to the wall at a line of small round tables. To my left a man with an enormous bald head was busy at his screen. To my right two men leaned towards each other and spoke in whispers.

I took out my laptop and sipped the coffee.

The men beside me were speaking English. The man on my left finished his emails and went away.

The man with his back to the wall was slim, nervous and Polish. He wore a cord jacket. A lawyer, perhaps, he spoke in broken English and I could pick up his entire narrative.

He worked for a law firm involved with IT and, as he put

it himself, they fucked him over. Apparently he was spending twelve hours a day working for very little money, and he was going over and back to London, sometimes every week, for many months without getting properly compensated.

It was all wearing him down. His health was suffering. But they wouldn't allow him even to buy into the company or they wouldn't give him a bonus.

So all this really pissed him off.

Even though I was close to them, they didn't bother hiding the conversation because I suppose they thought I didn't speak English. Or maybe because nobody cares about privacy anymore.

The man listening to him was stout, and looked about seventy. He wore a grey anorak and had a huge belly, a round face, and when he spoke I realised he was American.

He said he once worked in Afghanistan, in security companies.

'You ever think of doing something like that?' he asked. 'The people in Afghanistan are great, really great people. Yeah, it's a mess, sure, but fuck that, there's money to be made over there.'

The Polish man didn't look like he'd be much use in a security job in Butlins, never mind in Kabul. And he was more interested in laying out his stall. He obviously had a good package for the American.

He said he had information on all the IT companies in Poland. He knew what was being developed. He knew the games that were going to make millions in the next few years, even though they weren't even on the market yet. Games in development, he called them. He had been a CEO for a company that developed a particular game.

'The game was so good,' he said, 'that when they put a trial version on YouTube, they got over a million hits in one week. That's the kind of thing I'm talking about. I know these companies. I know the good ones, and I know what they have got.'

'So what do you want from me?' the American asked.

'Well, if you get in now,' doctor techie said, 'you can buy a majority of the shares in any of those companies and you can either support the development of the company to expand the product, or you can simply take the patent from them once you buy them out, and patent it for America and then it's yours to develop. There are two ways to go on this. But it's your choice.'

I was trying to avoid following the conversation too intensely, so I started thinking about a farmer in Cavan who died by moonlight. Just to distract myself.

A man who worked so hard that he could be heard at night in good weather, driving his tractor up and down the road, with a buckrake on the back, carrying hay bales from the big field to the hay shed in his back yard.

As he was reversing to lift the final bale, he drove close to the ditch, and the wheel got caught in a rut and the machine tipped over and pinned his lower body to the ground. He may have shouted for help but nobody heard him. So he died by the light of the moon. And years later his brother told me the story with tears in his eyes.

'He was mangled,' the brother said to me. 'You wouldn't see the like of it in Afghanistan.'

Not that many people in Cavan would know what a mangled body might look like in Afghanistan. But it's funny the various ways people talk about the dead. And the details they remember.

Sometimes people stand around outside a funeral home or in the back yard of a farmhouse, talking about some sycamore the dead man planted years earlier. Or how the woman made bread every day, or where she went on her bicycle for eggs in the old days when the children were young and one of them had the whooping cough.

By focusing on my Cavan memories I was able to keep the real world around me at bay. To keep my attention away from what was being cooked up at the next table. But my attention kept being drawn back to their conversation.

The American said he had to talk to his money man. So he set up a link on his computer. I kept my head down in my own screen hoping that no one spoke to me. It occurred to me that if a waiter asked me something in English then they would immediately realise I had understood every word. And they might not be too pleased. The American looked like he could be easily annoyed.

I had a ghoulish vision of myself stuck in the toilet while the American told me more about his job as a security boss in Afghanistan, all the while holding me by the throat.

'I can't let you go now,' he might say. 'You know too much.'

I scrolled down Facebook to see if Natasha had any nice icons posted, but I couldn't find her page. I scrolled through a mire of other self-serving posts by people I didn't know, but I couldn't keep my attention off my neighbours.

And now there were three of them. Two in the room beside me and another one on the screen from New York.

The American made the introductions.

'John,' he said, to the screen, 'this is Marek. Marek. This is John.'

He stuck his nose further into the screen.

'And Marek here could be useful to us, John. So I'm going to let you two guys talk it out for a few minutes and then we'll see where we are.'

Marek, thin as a whippet with golf-ball eyes, went through his pitch again about the information he had. And how he could finger the companies that were about to make money from their creative gaming software.

And the man on the screen listened and grunted, and at the end he just said, 'So … what can we do for you?'

Marek said how much money he wanted. How it would all be tied in with the delivery of the companies, and how he had his own company which was a real star, and how it got so many hits on the one week when they launched the trial version and that would be part of the package.

'How much is that?' the screen voice asked.

'That's 120K,' Marek said.

There was silence.

'OK,' the screen voice said at last.

And Marek said, 'Of course there would be initial expenses for gathering some of the detailed information. It's going to take time and some movement about the country. I would need to finalise some things with people.'

'So how much is that?'

Marek didn't put a figure on it.

And the screen voice said, 'You get that sorted with Steve.'

146

'Yes, John,' Steve said, 'I can handle that side of it.'

'Great,' Marek said.

'So we're good to go?' Steve asked. Like it was a question.

'All fine,' the screen said. 'It was nice talking to you.'

Steve closed the lid and the Voice from America was gone and the two boys tried to remain cool, and not over-excited, as they made small talk about the weather, Afghanistan, fucking women, being married and getting old.

It was over.

I was relieved.

But I needed to use the toilet before I left, which meant putting my computer in the rucksack, putting on my jacket, swinging the rucksack onto my shoulder and then edging past where they were sitting.

The American flashed a glance at me as I moved. I could feel the scan of his security eyes probing me.

And then the door to the toilets, not far from where we were all sitting, was locked. I tried but couldn't open it. I noticed a little keyboard beside the door on the wall and I knew I'd need to punch in a code. Which I didn't have.

Fuck it.

I would need to ask a waiter. But asking a waiter would draw attention to the fact that I was an English speaker.

So I left with a full bladder and headed home, to shut the door.

Not to Skype or phone the beloved. But just to sit on the toilet, and make coffee, and look out from the balcony and feel secure in my own little world.

147

The privatisation of religious faith is its own downfall. And more and more, as days turned into weeks, I'd spent less time on the streets, or in the churches, and more time sitting in the apartment, drinking vodka or watching Netflix.

According to medieval monks there was an illness beneath depression. It was not depression but it was close to it. Deeper. Called despondency. It was the ability to care for nothing, know nothing, feel nothing, do nothing. Because there was nothing.

And I felt it. And I was reading Beckett too, *Malone Dies* and *Murphy*, random paragraphs here and there and thinking maybe this despondency virus is still on the go. Maybe the monks in the deserts knew more about the mind than we care to admit.

I finally spoke to the beloved. She phoned as I was on the street.

She was in the front room at home in Arigna, with a Polish man who lives in Drumshanbo. He was cleaning the chimney for her. I told her it was minus 5.

She asked me was I wearing a scarf.

I said I wasn't.

She said that the chimney sweep said I must wear a scarf at all times.

'He knows what it's like in Warsaw, and he says you need a scarf.'

'OK.'

148   So I went looking for a clothes shop.

I went into the arcade beside the train station, and began looking around one shop after another on the second floor.

At first I was only looking for scarves. But then I began looking at coats, because the anorak I had brought from Ireland had never been sufficient. It was too small. And the other shoppers were wearing coats as big and as fat as duvets, down below their knees. And scarves.

A young salesman in a blue suit saw me come in the door; he spoke English and was very good at bamboozling me about what I wanted and telling me how well I would look in this or that coat, so that in the end I was so confused I gave him €150 for the coat he called perfect.

He could have sold me a bicycle and an umbrella as well. He was good.

I went off with the coat in a big fancy carrier bag with the shop name on both sides. But in the apartment I discovered that the coat was too tight.

And how, I wondered, looking at myself in the mirror, could I have been so stupid as to buy something with buttons rather than a zip.

The following day I found a much better option by accident, in a second-hand shop: an anorak that went down below my knees, and had a zip which closed in under my chin, and it had a hood, and it was only twelve euros. And I even found a scarf as well.

That evening I put the insulation layer from the expensive coat into the cheap one and it fitted perfectly.

For days afterwards I would cheer myself up just by looking at it hanging in the wardrobe, and I would run my fingers over it, like a girl with a new dress. All this and a scarf too.

So maybe they will soften the numb leg, I hoped, calm the flashing eye and diminish the pain when I breathe in cold air.

But they didn't.

I struggled one day to get as far as the concert hall. I was wearing the new coat, feeling cosy on the streets, but still I couldn't walk. My feet felt like lead. And I had developed a persistent dry cough. I was breathless all the time. Still, I got to the concert hall, and was calm and relaxed and got a lovely seat on the corner of the first balcony.

It was a cello competition. All the musicians were young boys and girls. Each one was introduced by an elderly man in a dinner jacket and white dickie bow. He gave long speeches before each performance, and then left the stage with a limp and a shoe that squeaked.

The young musician began.

A Japanese boy played a Haydn sonata with the orchestra.

Melodious. Consoling. Welcoming. Comforting me like the coat. In the apartment that night I found the music on Spotify and played it over and over again.

And I kept going back to the concert hall every day for more music. The cello competition went on for two weeks. It became my church above all churches.

The Church of the Vibrating Christ.

I sat through a sonata by Lutosławski one evening, mesmerised by a boy wrestling with his cello, on the stage, before the orchestra, and the conductor with long hands and arms trying to control the boy's passion as the boy stretched himself in a black T-shirt and trousers, a black scarf and jacket, with his eyes closed.

He bent over the cello as if it were his beloved. As if he was sheltering a child from all the ugly things in life. And he'd sometimes draw the bow out long, and sideways, across the strings, so that his back arched, and his body leaned away from the instrument and his eyes opened, and he looked not at the audience, but into some place between the notes, as if he, like me, could feel some Christ vibrating in the moment. As if he was experiencing the music passively and was being lacerated in ecstasy by it.

'Christ is the silence between the notes,' I whispered.

And there I was doing it all again. Praying. Even at a cello concert I couldn't stop.

In his cello music the musician was releasing himself from all the pain of being mortal. An elegant letting go, in every note. Inhabiting an astonishing silence between the notes as he became more present, more alive, more real before my eyes with every phrase of music that issued from the strings.

Round glasses with
a wide bridge

U p on the first balcony I spilled a discreet tear of joy from the side of my eye wrapped in a silence of my own making. Without being able to write, or articulate anything on the writing screen, the days in Warsaw had become painful, debilitating, and they'd seemed like a prefiguring of something terrible on the horizon.

Writer's block can be more devastating than people imagine. It can indicate the opening of a deep despondency, choking creativity with desire and anger; it is an asphyxiation in the dead zone of non-being, dragging the victim away from the here and now.

And when despondency has destroyed the ability to sing, tell, speak, or write any more stories there are only two alternatives: take refuge in a psychiatric hospital and close the door, or lean on someone else's work for consolation.

For me the refuge in those moments of despair was Beckett, and music, so that at night I wrapped around me the blades of music like a comfort blanket and as I watched the musician on stage I felt that his agony was my own.

My leg was very sore that night. And the flashing at the corner of my eye came with the regularity of a strobe light pulsing all through the dark hours until dawn when I rose and brushed my teeth. Now there was blood in the basin. Something going wrong with the gums too perhaps. I looked in the mirror and laughed. There's no end to these failures, I thought.

But just as my heart had emptied a few days earlier, letting go all hope and joy, so one morning it filled up again.

154 Hope and joy flowed back into every chamber of my heart as if the blood itself was flowing more freely. And it may have been because my leg too felt warmer and more alive. And I rinsed out my mouth and picked up my clothes from where they lay in a bundle on the white-tiled floor. I costumed up as complete and thorough as any astronaut heading for a space walk, in anorak, leggings, scarf and hat, and went out the door and off downtown before this new hope petered away.

I was heading for the Orthodox Cathedral of Mary Magdalene.

Over the bridge, along the edge of the zoo with its parkland of bare-frosted trees. And then, just as I was about to go up the steps of the cathedral I realised I couldn't do it.

Fuck it. I just couldn't go in.

I passed it by and headed for the underground.

I walked through the subway passage, which reeked of urine, to an escalator which brought me back up to ground level on the far side of the street and I moved towards the gleaming glass walls of Starbucks and the promise of hot coffee, sweet buns and the warm glow of human faces in the cosy café.

On the following few mornings I repeated the trip, sitting in Starbucks across from the cathedral, as if being that close was enough, though I yearned to go inside.

My mood went up and down with increasing drama. One morning I would head for the cathedral. The next morning because of fatigue I just went as far as the shop on the corner beside the apartment. And there were days when I struggled to get out of bed at all, with a stiff back, numb legs and a new pain in my left arm, like a knot of muscle deep inside which refused to unlock.

I became breathless more often. I felt the freezing fog sink into my lungs as if sandpaper was scraping the insides of my throat.

I found it difficult to rise and get to the desk, with a little glass of kefir from the fridge, and an enormous pear from the worktop and a mug of tea. And almost every day I would open Facebook and look for some cheer, but never find it.

On Facebook they just chatted away in their own worlds. In their happy mornings, about their party nights. About wedding days and anniversaries. About photos taken on the Great Wall of China or on the streets near Times Square. At the pool in Spain or a barbecue in Bali. Or in the back garden of a semi-detached in Mullingar.

155

I looked at Facebook as one would look into a pool of water to see if there might be a fish playing a violin at the bottom of it. But there never was. So I closed it down and took an icon of the Mother of Jesus out of my briefcase and stood it up on a ledge beside the bed, where I could see it from the desk. Because when I looked out the window, I knew the real world would never offer me any magic that could be described as a fish with a violin.

Sometimes I walked in the sleet across Saski Park as far as Old Town where I had one more latte in Costa Coffee and pushed further into the cold air up Nowy Świat, and then all the way up town to the Jewish cemetery on the other side of John Paul Avenue.

I moved about the graves and the beautiful monuments and sculptural forms as if I were searching for an old friend in the dead leaves.

One day I heard children from Israel laughing and joking as they held hands and took photographs of gravestones, while security men with machine guns and balaclavas watched over them at a little distance.

But in the end I went back to Praga, the district across the river from Old Town, because something called me. I had my coffee in Starbucks, gazing out the window at the onion dome, and finally crossed through the subway and emerged at the Orthodox cathedral once again and walked up the steps.

Something was sucking me down a sinkhole.

I spent an hour in the dark interior, standing with the incense in my nostrils, a golden intensity around the saintly heads of icons. They grew warm inside me, like the shock of strong coffee. Still listening for a fish to play the music. And sensing that I was close to that moment when the veil gets torn asunder and from another world a chink of light slips into this.

Alone at night, I dropped words in the silence, like pebbles in a well, like Beckett on a park bench, and other times I spoke as if I were talking to my beloved.

It was madness.

I was talking to myself. I was breaking down.

When the beloved appeared on FaceTime I told her none of this. Instead I brought her up-to-date on every optician's window I had seen. On the shape and size of glasses in a dozen shops along the arcades and shopping malls. And though all of that was true, nonetheless it was also a complex fabrication of betrayal.

The only further interruption in this isolated dark was when the spectacles appeared. I was sitting at a table on the street, with a coffee, near the Royal Palace. It was the morning after I had finally managed to walk up the steps of the Orthodox cathedral and enter it.

The square opened before me, a pedestrian area leading to Old Town. I was actually planning another trip to the Cathedral of Mary Magdalene when I noticed, at the far end of the square, an optician's sign I had not seen before.

I walked across the square, to the edge of the first little street that leads to an old twelfth-century church managed by Jesuits, at which point I looked in the shop window.

It didn't even look like an optician's shop. The facade was medieval, like the other buildings, and only a small sign above the door revealed that it was a shop.

In the window there were a few pairs of glasses.

I looked in.

An elderly woman was sitting at a desk inside. She had grey hair in a bun and round spectacles. She was about my age. Her little round glasses sat perfectly on the bridge of her nose.

That's them, I thought. Those are the glasses I need.

I went inside.

158   I explained what I wanted. Round glasses with a wide bridge for the nose.

'Something like you are wearing,' I suggested.

She smiled. Then she went to a desk and pulled out several drawers, picking out a few pairs of spectacles, examining each and throwing them back. Finally she got the ones I wanted.

'These are like mine,' she said, handing them over.

They fitted perfectly over my ears.

She had brown eyes.

'They look well on you,' I said.

'Thank you,' she replied. 'Will you take them?'

'Yes.'

She tapped in a few figures on a pocket calculator.

'It will be a hundred euros.'

I went off for an hour, while she put glass in the frames to match my prescription. When I returned she had them wrapped up in a little red box.

I paid with a plastic credit card. Checked myself in the mirror. And went away to the Orthodox cathedral to give thanks.

Because I was alone for four weeks and had lain in the same bed with grey sheets, and sat on the same balcony every morning as it froze or rained, I had found completion.

There was something wrong with my health but I couldn't put a finger on it. Instead of going to a doctor, or considering it rationally, I was swallowed by emotions which ill-health was producing. I became despondent, and convinced myself that the only flicker of hope in my life was religious – the glow of that old lantern of magical thinking.

159

I loitered around the Roman Catholic churches long enough for the old swagger of clerics and wizened nuns to get up my nose, and then in desperation I went looking for an alternative, which was what the Orthodox cathedral offered me. It was unfamiliar enough to be exotic. Familiar enough to feel like home.

One night I went to the cinema and saw the wrong movie. It was late when the movie ended. From Arkadia I walked through temperatures of minus 14 on my way back to the apartment. My ribcage really hurt by now. The knot in my left arm was frightening me.

I needed to take a tram. But I stood too long at a tram stop waiting for a tram that didn't come. I stomped my feet and watched the other night wanderers from inside my cowled hood.

But at least I was wearing my new spectacles; as if they were the only thing that constituted what was me.

To use the florid language of fourth-century monks in the deserts of Egypt, I was possessed by the discomfiting silence of God, the exquisite indifference of the cosmos.

I had long ago stopped believing in all that wonder, but here I was again infatuated by the erotic frills of divine liturgies, incense and candles. Yet again I was locked into a monastic cell of glorious solitude on the eighth floor of an indifferent Soviet apartment block.

I was self-sufficient. There was no one I needed outside that room to complete my joy. That was betrayal.

160

Solitude rather than another human person became the lure that closed off intimacy with my beloved.

A month in Warsaw may not seem like much. But as a journey inwards it had been sufficient to make my despondency complete. I'd wallowed in a secret garden of the heart, from which I had excluded all else: the world and all its beauties; the strangers, friends and enemies that make us who we are.

They were all banished. It didn't augur well for the tattered heart.

If only it had snowed, that might have cheered me up or drawn me out of the solid self I was enclosed in, like a prison, during that grim winter month.

Because snow should be a certainty in Warsaw.

It's not like Leitrim, where every year I hoped, and waited, day after day for snow to come, especially near Christmas.

For years I would look at the sky in Leitrim during December and convince myself that snow was coming. Perhaps it was already snowing somewhere else.

It will come from the sky, I'd say, from out of the clouds on a dark evening, soon, when the farmers are leaning into the wind with fodder on their backs for cattle that stand in waterlogged fields.

It will snow when the woodcutter takes the chainsaw and ladder to the tip of the last tree in the forest, I would think, on Christmas Eve, as his children wait on the roadside shouting, 'Daddy! Daddy! Don't let it fall out on the road, there's a car coming.'

And maybe it would snow when the women were about to turn the ignition in their cars, and head home after a night of fizzy waters and orange juices in the pub, with husbands as useless as mules.

And when they were about to lie down at night, and they peeped out through the curtains to make sure the outside light in the yard was off, it would snow, and they would see it, magical and wonderful, and they would be tempted to wake the children, with excited whispers, saying, 'Look out the window! It's snowing now!'

That's the way I imagined it somewhere, always, and my daughter would say, 'But Daddy, you wait for it every year, but it never snows.'

I'd say nothing, because she would not yet understand that I needed something to believe in.

Now that there is no more Holy Communion, and the crib gathers dust in the attic, and the clergy talk endless gobbledegook, I am stranded in a miserable rain, in a flooded field, in a wet and indifferent Leitrim Christmas, and my last remaining hope is in the possibility of snow.

Is it any wonder I would want to go to Warsaw.

Inside the door of a shopping mall in Mullingar a group of teenagers in Santa hats were murdering 'Silent Night' one year, and a man sat outside the ladies' toilet, with a child in a buggy. There was an office party in a nearby bar, and a young woman emerged and noticed the man waiting with the buggy.

'Will you come in and have a drink?' she asked.

'No,' the man said, 'I'm just waiting for the wife; she's still in the toilet.'

Beside the buggy was a red box that contained a 32-inch LCD screen, or so the box proclaimed. The child in the buggy slept. The man waited, staring at the box, like he too was a child, waiting for Christmas morning.

I asked him did he think there might be snow.

He grimaced, and said, 'Not a chance.'

On the street outside, a man was having an argument with a parking meter. I explained that parking was free until two o'clock.

'But if you put in some euros now, you can buy the time from two until four,' I suggested.

He was impressed by such intelligence in a machine.

I asked him did he think it would snow.

'My friend,' he declared, 'I couldn't care a monkey's uncle what the weather does, because come Sunday morning I'm off to Alicante.'

And then, finally, a Romanian woman in a long purple dress asked me for money. I placed a two-euro coin in her plastic cup.

Then she took the coin from the cup and held it up, saying, 'Please. Coffee.'

She wanted me to take back the money and go into Subway and buy her a hot drink.

'They not like me to go inside shop,' she said.

I left the €2 in her cup and went to the shop and got her the coffee.

'What is your name?' she asked, when I returned.

I told her, and then inquired for her name, which she gave me.

A green headscarf covered her black hair and she pushed her face close to mine, with the ease and brass of a skilled beggar. Her eyes were brown and her skin as smooth as almonds, and her lips were a foggy blue and as moist as a sloe in November.

In the distance, a waltz was playing; beneath the arch to the car park a portly gent in a brown leather jacket, with oily black hair, sallow skin, a wart on his nose and a big grey moustache, played his accordion.

'Are you with him?' I wondered.

'My father,' she said.

I asked her did she think it would snow.

'Of course it will snow,' she said, confident and happy.

'Maria! Maria!' her father called out, eyeing the coffee.

She placed her hand on her breast and said, 'In my country it always snows.'

And with that certainty I often went east in the winter, just for snow. I went to Krakow and Bucharest and Warsaw. But in 2018 it did not snow in Warsaw. And to make things worse, while I was away, it began snowing in Ireland.

164

The Irish snowstorm

I couldn't believe it when the beloved had described it. In Leitrim the back yard was covered white. The fields all about had blended with the roads and laneways. Only the ditches stuck up out of the white blanket.

She was smiling into the computer screen. I could see the flames in the stove behind her. The cat was in.

Fuck this, I'd thought. Fuck it.

There was a snowstorm raging in Ireland and it was predicted to get worse. A beast from the east was leaving roads impossible to travel, closing down airports and sweeping across the roofs of the houses.

And all this happened when I was in Warsaw. Me who loves snow. Me who would cross the Alps to see snow. There I was on rainy streets, and it was snowing in Ireland.

Fuck that!

I wasn't just frustrated. I was infuriated. It seemed to crown a miserable month. It seemed to be the perfect end to a disastrous retreat.

I needed to get home.

I made contact with the beloved again the next morning and said I had booked a flight home, and we chatted about the details and she warned me that the snow was going to be very heavy the following day.

'Don't worry about that,' I said. 'I need to get home.'

So early on Wednesday I went to the airport. It was the last day of February, 2018. And my fears were confirmed. All fights to Dublin had been cancelled. There would be no more until Monday morning.

166   But I needed to get home, to see Leitrim, so when I saw a flight to Liverpool on the departures board I went to a Ryanair counter, showed him my ticket for Dublin and asked could I get on the Liverpool flight.

'But Liverpool is not in Ireland,' the agent said.

'I know that,' I replied, 'but I will take the flight if it's open.'

It was. And I took it.

Arriving in England from Europe seemed different since the Brexit referendum. Usually I'd expect to see a few gentle signs for passport control with EU flags. But the signs in Liverpool were stark.

UK Border, they proclaimed, in bold red, white and blue. As if Britian was no longer part of Europe.

And maybe I looked suspicious, because I was taken aside as I walked through customs.

'Can you come this way, sir?' the lady officer asked.

'And do you have any cigarettes today?' she asked, pointing at my luggage.

'I don't smoke,' I confessed, which I thought was funny.

She wasn't amused. But she let me pass.

In Liverpool I measured out the day in mugs of coffee. And on one occasion the wireless pay machine wasn't working at the cash desk and I had no sterling.

'I have only Polish money,' I joked, but the man just stared back at me. He wasn't amused.

It was a long day, in a desolate arrivals hall.

Eventually a flight to Cork appeared on the departures board, and I promised myself I would be on it if it took off.

It did. And I was. At about seven o'clock that evening. Except that when we got close to Cork, the pilot announced that the airport was closed because of a blizzard. So he flew to Shannon. Which didn't amuse a farmer from Clare who had phoned the wife to say he was heading for Cork.

'She's after driving three hours in the snow,' he said, 'to pick me up in Cork, and now you want me to phone her and tell her I'm in Shannon, fifteen minutes from my front door.'

I had booked a hotel in Cork, and seats on the morning train to Dublin and the afternoon train to Carrick-on-Shannon. But in Shannon I learned that the trains were cancelled.

However, there was a bus stop outside the airport where people were gathering for a connection to Galway. So I hopped on that when it came and was in Galway by midnight. It was snowing heavily by now. But I found a wonderful night porter in the Meyrick, who got me a room and said he could bring me a pot of coffee in the morning at 5 a.m.

Which he did, and I went off to find the 6 a.m. bus for Sligo.

I waited outside at the stop for half an hour but no bus came, and I presumed that too had been cancelled.

There was, on the other hand, a train warming up on the platform of the station behind me.

'Where's that going?' I wondered, and someone said it was heading for Dublin. So I got a ticket from the machine, jumped on board and hoped to get as far as Athlone. Now I was getting really close to Leitrim, although the roads from Athlone to Leitrim would be impossible to negotiate.

But before arriving in Athlone I phoned a friend in Mullingar who was out early delivering the daily vegetables to nursing homes in the county and he said the N4 and the N52 to Tullamore were both open.

'Stay on the train until Tullamore,' he suggested. Which I did, and had a fine breakfast in the Bridge Hotel as I waited for the beloved, who had agreed to risk driving from Leitrim.

The foyer was busy. People with seriously ill relatives in the local hospital were checking into the hotel because they couldn't go home. Ciaran Mullooly, the television news journalist, was in his working anorak with headphones on his ears chatting with his cameraman. And as I looked out across the snow-covered patio seats from the breakfast room,

I saw my beloved's Citroën crunching through the snow-covered street towards the hotel door.

'I'm safe,' I whispered.

And grateful later that evening for my home, a fire and a glass of whiskey.

And grateful too for all the people out there, clearing the snow, driving the ambulances and fixing the electrical lines.

And grateful to the Ryanair staff, the Galway bus driver, the night porter in the Meyrick and the multitude of others who had made my journey from Poland to Leitrim possible.   169

I had stood in freezing fog waiting at a tram stop in Poland on Wednesday morning with my bags. Now I was back in the hills above Lough Allen, thirty-six hours later, in the company of my beloved, wondering, as I often do, how does she put up with me.

OLD HORNPIPES

The fish in the fridge

I remember a few years earlier, in 2012, hearing the news about the death of Savita Halappanavar from septicaemia in a Galway maternity hospital, because she was refused a medical termination based on the fact that the foetus displayed a heartbeat, and as a nurse explained to the dying woman: 'This is a Catholic country, dear.'

I was in bed when I heard that story on the radio. I was still recovering from colitis and I just went back to sleep. But even when I got up later in the day I was only half awake. I ate my dinner with closed eyes, watched *Homeland* that evening, read short stories on the train to Dublin the following day, and all the while, for two days, I might as well have been still asleep.

And as the week went on I couldn't bear the evening news. I couldn't bear the world anymore. I couldn't bear the upset in people's voices on radio talk shows.

I felt it was raining in the house. There were big damp clouds in the hot press. It rained on the kitchen table and on the hallstand. It never stopped raining. The bathroom was flooded. The bed floated on rising water.

By the end of the week I was so immobilised that I began to wish for the Great Silence. I'd sit in the armchair, the one I took from my mother's house, where she sat waiting for her ending, and I'd sit alone.

When other people hugged me there was a distance between us. I didn't grasp them with any zest. My body behaved politely but full of shame. It was as if we were in parallel universes, as if the sun was shining on them all the time and I was standing in the rain.

I saw the woman who died in Galway, Savita in a white dress, dancing on YouTube. She seemed intensely alive, while my clothes felt like the drapery of the grave, and the people around me in the supermarkets were like the sleeping damned in an underworld they didn't even try to resist.

I felt like the man whose fridge stood outside an old house for over a decade until he opened the door and found a dead rat, and in the freezer box a fish that had turned to liquid. The smell was intense, but he knew what it was because ten years earlier he had argued with his girlfriend about who should clean that same fish. She said that he should at least clean the fridge. He never did. They fell apart. The fridge remained intact, silent and frozen through ten winters, until he opened it again and discovered what human beings are capable of.

And it's funny how no matter what terrible detail is in the dying, the rest of us continue to forget.

I knew some corners of Fermanagh where human beings were executed and where the trees now look just so beautiful that I often wonder was I dreaming all that blood in the long ago. But I suppose that's what the politicians hope for: that we will forget and they can continue to do nothing.

But I didn't want to do nothing, like I always do. So I drove to Dublin on 17 November to be part of the vigil for the woman who died in Galway.

There were thousands of women, walking quietly in the rain. Quietly moving towards the parliament. Pushing buggies. Holding each other's arms. Moving through the streets with a silent dignity that reminded me of Máirtín Ó Direáin's poem about the dignity of grief, 'Dínit an Bhróin'.

175

And I felt that the shame in me was lifting. I was not immobile anymore. At last, at long last, I was doing something; I was walking with them.

During that demonstration about the death of Savita, everyone was given a small candle, which we lit at the end of the march, and when it was over I put the stub of the candle in my pocket.

The day after that Dublin march in 2012 I placed the candle on the shelf of my father's bookcase that stood in the corner of my studio.

By 2018 that bookcase had become an icon corner, and the shelves were full of sacred images and objects, and the candle happened to be there as well. It seemed at home with the saints, and the chalice and the prayer rope and the golden oil lamps.

On the last Sunday morning before the referendum to repeal the eighth amendment I lit the candle once again, and watched the flickering light illuminate the icon of the Great Mother so that her golden halo shimmered in the morning light. I wanted to stand with a cause I believed was about justice. And I also wanted to reclaim my Christian faith. And the strange thing which I couldn't quite understand, and still don't, is that for me the referendum was a moment in which I could both reclaim my faith again and also stand for justice. Both in the same time became linked in a way that 176 undermined the simplistic moral certainties of Christian churches.

The bitter despondency that had dogged my soul bleakly all through my time in Warsaw was gone. I was for something, at last, rather than against everything. And while I knew I was for repealing the eighth amendment, I also felt that something had loosened in my heart, some despondent energy had been unblocked, and I felt a sense of permission again, to pray, even if I was praying for the success of the Yes side in the referendum.

Coming off the fence

I t's not that I had ever thought much about abortion. For a man it's almost impossible to hold any view with ease and my default position for years would have been like many other men: democracy impels us to accept the full autonomy of women on the matter.

So what's wrong with that?

I suppose it's a fine example of sitting on the fence. It's a tolerance which is never quite substantiated by men's involvement in the various causes or issues affecting women's right to choose. When it boils down to how you get your pills, men tend to think, well, it's not really for me to be sorting that out.

What became different in the 2018 referendum was that men began to take on board the fact that this was an issue of equality in law, and it mattered for democracy.

And it's interesting that the vast majority of males coming out of voting booths who were questioned said that they voted yes not on the moral issue, but on the basis of the woman's right to choose.

Six years earlier the human tragedy of Savita's life had clarified in many people's minds the need to sort out all the medical law in Ireland that was affecting women.

But personally I didn't do anything about it. I was still morally lazy enough to see it as someone else's issue. And I might have gone on through the time of the referendum campaign assuring anyone that I was voting yes, without ever having done much else about the matter.

But one day during April, I was in Cavan to get the Skoda serviced and, with an hour to spare before the appointed time, I drove up to the car park of the Kilmore Hotel. I took out my phone and placed it on the dashboard. Then, without any preparation, I made a short video; I talked for a few minutes about the rights of women to make choices about their own bodies, no matter how much anyone else agreed or disagreed.

As it happened, when I went home that evening and sat down at the television, the first thing that came up on Netflix was a documentary about Medjugorje. And it was so beautiful in its sense of hope and healing and love that I got caught up in it.

I went to bed and dreamed that my smartphone turned to mush and I lost my clothes and I got put up in a strange hotel. Naked, I had to share a room with others, but when I went into the room there were two dead people, one sitting by the bed looking at me, the other with a white gauze over her face, her eyes bulging through the gauze as she too stared in my direction.

And she began moving towards me across the room, saying, 'Where is your child, where is your child?'

I woke distressed.

But it crossed my mind that if I, as a man in his sixties, was having dreams like that just because I was conflicted about abortion, what effect was the referendum having on women who were trying at that very moment to cope with unwanted pregnancies, fatal foetal abnormalities or the consequences of a rape that had never been named.

How could I begin to understand the vast landscape of hurt and wound that was out there in Ireland, and which I had not bothered to wonder about.

One night when the beloved was staying in Dublin because of an early morning meeting, I went to the kitchen and ate a banana. I filled a glass of water from the tap and returned to bed. I finished half the water and fell asleep and dreamed I was cutting up my mother's body and packing it neatly into a suitcase.

Then again I woke suddenly, my arm across the edge of the bed, the upturned glass of water lying on the duvet and the bedclothes soaking wet.

I finished editing the video on 16 April. But I still slipped into churches, and lit candles on side altars and stood staring at the sanctuary lamp.

I whispered prayers to the Great Mother, the icon in my studio, but I began to pray a new prayer, and to sing a new song.

I was praying that the Yes side might win.

It didn't seem like a coherent position, considering the clarity of various Catholic bishops and commentators on the radio.

But I sent the video to the Together for Yes, Leitrim website and they posted it public, and in the following week over 150,000 people viewed it.

As the campaign moved onwards towards the referendum date I became glued to the television every evening watching debates about the issue.

180 *The Pat Kenny Show* hosted a final debate on the eve of the ballot. They asked a number of people for and against to make simple two-minute video clips stating their position. These were peppered into the programme.

They contacted me and I agreed with enthusiasm to do another video clip.

The following afternoon a film crew arrived at my studio; the filming took half an hour.

I spoke directly to the camera and I quoted the gospel where it says that we should not judge others. I said that nobody should try to impose the law of Christ with the sword of Caesar. That was it.

The cup of tea
with toast

I often regretted that I could not stay in the church. I admired the sacrifices good priests had made over the years, forgetting their comforts, living without the tenderness and joy of a companion, and devoting themselves to the care of others.

I have known priests who spent their entire days ministering to the sick, the elderly, the bereaved and the homeless.

But what triumphed in the official church during the referendum campaign was a voice of righteousness and authority.

The eighth amendment was crafted out of a peculiarly clerical kind of unease – that women can't be trusted to do good.

Women who faced the catastrophe of abortion, alone in a far-off country, away from their families and parents, were in truth only trying to cope. Yet the bishops told parents to shut them out, close the door in their faces and let them go to England and to hell.

Just as the hierarchy had previously told the nation to shut out gay families, arguing that their intimate acts of affection were criminal, and that the love in their hearts was dysfunctional.

But if they shut out gay people, and shut out the divorced, and shut out the poor, and shut out women, then who would they have left to share their good news with?

For me the good news was that human beings were infinitely loveable and always capable of forgiveness.

Although it's not to clerics I would go to now, for forgiveness. Rather I would turn to women, and those who have been wounded, isolated and judged by the fierce annunciations of a judgemental hierarchy – and beg forgiveness from them, for myself and my brothers in the lofty ranks of the hierarchy.

Because I am truly sorry that the church I once belonged to treated women with such unmerciful judgement, and that I did so little to support their plight over the years.

The referendum was passed. The eighth amendment was taken out of the Constitution. It didn't feel to me like either side had won the moral high ground. It just felt like the world had moved on.

I was quiet for a long while afterwards. I stoked the range. Sat burning small logs that I cut from two trees which had blown down in the storms of spring.

I'd woken up at about 4 p.m. on the day after the heart attack. There was a grey light falling on the stainless steel instruments in an empty surgical room. A solitary nurse in light blue trousers and top, still wearing her mask, was watching a screen where a thin line indicated the nuances of my heart's rhythm.

I had a stent. The blood was flowing freely. A cup of tea with toast was sitting on a tray at the foot of my bed. From this day onwards I have only one destiny, I thought. To give thanks. To sing my gratitude to the world. To the doctors and nurses. To the paramedics who got to me within nine minutes of me placing the call for help.

The only problem was that I didn't know how to give thanks, or where to express gratitude, or to whom. And I wondered about it for weeks. Walking around the house for little ten-minute sessions, and trying to remember not to lift bales of turf briquettes from the boot of the car, and idling in bed late in the mornings, and keeping my eye on any appointments with the doctor, or at the hospital.

But I wasn't depressed. And it amazed me. In previous years, after being burned out and hospitalised with colitis, I had stared at the lake for a year feeling emasculated and broken by sudden illness, and depression set in like cement. So I would have been prepared for a long winter.

I had even heard of men suffering weeks of weeping and lethargy after the inviolability of their hearts were undermined by the insertion of one or many stents.

'I should be depressed,' I told the beloved, 'but I'm not.'

It was a miracle to be cheerful in Leitrim during any winter. The county becomes a dark and bleak landscape of sitka trees and empty fields and old rusting sheds. In winter the cat would sometimes sit on the sill, inside, looking out, and I would say, 'Don't do that, pussy. Don't look out, you will only depress yourself.'

And then the relentless damp of winter in Leitrim turns the woodlands into such a swamp that by March I often met frogs the size of myself among the trees. Those were bleak years when I'd open my eyes and struggle to get out of bed.

But after the stent, I had no such depression. And by March I began to notice a light in the sky, a luminous blue covering the heavens. The sky was beautiful. The weather had changed. The rain had finally stopped.

184

We had a wonderful spring.

The lake was blue. Seven long miles of Lough Allen's lovely waters glowed like the Virgin Mary's blouse, and the mountains beyond were vivid in every fold and crevice where the streams cascaded down towards the lake, and the little white houses near Dowra glistened in the distance like a necklace of white pebbles.

To the north the windmills were as small as toothpicks, and the hills of Fermanagh were blurred in a grey haze as lovely as any summer heatwave.

I went into the garden, and stood beneath branches of beech leaf, yellow and copper. I was encountering an invisible world that surfaces only occasionally and which makes all the dark days in Leitrim worthwhile. My depression was gone. My usual winter melancholy had evaporated.

What was up?

I was so happy that I put honey on my porridge one morning, like a child. And Miss Peabody, the black and white cat, appeared happy too. I could see her prancing along the top of the wooden fence, with a cocky swagger as if she thought she were invisible to the birds.

I stood long enough in the garden to allow the blue of sky and lake seep into my bones.

I was a bit afraid of getting back into the pool but one morning I took the risk and went to the leisure centre in Carrick-on-Shannon.

185

I had lost a lot of confidence about parading naked after the stent, but nonetheless, I slipped into togs and swimming cap, showered, stood for a moment on the tiles at the pool's edge, and then descended the ladder into the water as if descending into a lake. I didn't swim. I just stood there, in the water, clutching the ladder.

The pool was almost empty – only me and a lifeguard, who was perched on a high chair at the far end of the pool. There was no sign of the ladies who usually come in the morning for aerobics, waving their hands in the air and swivelling around in unison like seals imprisoned in an American aquarium.

I didn't want to go into the sauna, in case it was too hot and affected my blood pressure, but I sat alone in the cloudy steamroom, gazing through the glass door at the pool where an elderly lady dipped her toe delicately into the water before lunging forward into a breaststroke. She was like a familiar bird. I realised I'd been watching her for years.

She moved up and down the pool for ten minutes looking from side to side with the gentility of a lazy duck. She too must have been wondering where everybody was.

Then she left and went into the sauna. The surface of the pool regained the composure of glass, the sunlight through high windows slanting across the still water.

And she didn't linger in the sauna either. Maybe she too has a stent, I thought. Maybe someday soon I will swim like her, as lazy as a bird crossing the sky. I could see her again when she emerged from the sauna, her deck shoes squeaking as she made her way to the changing rooms, their flip-flop sound fading eventually into the distance.

Everything felt different from the previous year, when the campaign to repeal the eighth amendment began.

Now there was silence. Real silence, creeping into my heart. A singular moment of delicious emptiness, and I knew I had changed. My heart was recovered. Although I hadn't even realised it had been sick through all those years of melancholy.

Paper lanterns

My mother used to leave jugs of water on the table on All Souls' Eve so that when the wounded in the other world came visiting they would be comforted by water. And since she died I often say that she is just beyond my fingertips.

I know there is a deficit of rational thinking in both her devotions around All Souls' Night and my way of expressing how close she is to the surface of my memory. But I am a writer and I use metaphor all the time. It is the tool of my trade. We shape ourselves and our universe in metaphors. To live without them is, at least for writers, impossible.

We are so completely infused with sign and symbol, and our language is so constructed to carry metaphor, that it is fair to say, as Rilke did, that the human being is a symbol that reaches perfection in death.

It wasn't difficult for me as a child to figure out that water in Ireland was the most powerful symbol of all – a symbol of hope in the face of anxiety, hunger, illness, and even death.

Holy water stretches beyond the threshold of the visible world, into the shadows where we are all heading.

Every county in Ireland is peppered with holy wells – dark pools rising from the rocks below, shaded sanctuaries where spiders thrive, sheltered by old stone walls that keep the wind at bay. And sometimes bushes of rag and bandage or holy medals stand nearby, proclaiming cures and blessings received at the well of spring water.

In ecological terms Ireland is a plentiful mother who nurtures humans as well as wild animals and every form of vegetation. The mountains and valleys are full of her name, and water is her elixir, its nourishment oozing out from bogs and swamps and mountain streams. The white goddess is a hidden presence everywhere, in lakes, off-shore islands and in the May bushes that flourish from Antrim to Kerry, where the curved hills are known as the Breasts of Anú.

And when the Christians first set foot on Erin with their new-fangled images of a masculine God, it was water that their monks sang about. They chanted their praise of a 'God' who comes like 'living water to a dry, weary land'.

On 23 June 2018 I stood in a field and plucked a tiny yellow flower that had four petals. The smoke of St John's Eve bonfires was rising from various locations along the slopes of the mountain across the lake. We were moving deeper into summer and the Great Mother Earth was wide awake and singing in her fecundity.

I went into my studio and began to pray. To count the knots on a prayer rope. To whisper chants of ancient monks who had lived in the deserts of Egypt 1,500 years ago, and in Ireland since the sixth century – on islands in Fermanagh and Cavan, in the valleys and along the coastline in Donegal, and all through the west of Ireland, and down as far as the Skellig Rock. This was once an island of monks not unlike those in the deserts of Egypt. They were warriors of interior space, travellers in the psyche, storytellers, book binders, iconographers and psychotherapists who parsed the destructive force of the psyche into demons, and went to battle with them in a crucible of silence. And Europe was imagined out of the foundations that they had left in their wake.

189

But it's difficult to re-imagine from the stones of old monastic sites what exactly it might have looked like when the cloisters echoed with Greek chanting or when the stones were a blaze of colour and iconic narratives decked the sanctuary walls.

I have walked among the fallen stones sometimes, scattered through meadows, and seen the ruined huts and prayer halls on islands and lonely places off the western seaboard.

And although I can't imagine what it was like in Ireland twelve hundred years ago, I have been to Electric Picnic and the Body and Soul festival enough times to know that warriors, shamanic ritual and the power of myth still grip young people's imagination.

I went to the Festival of the Fires on Uisneach Hill in Westmeath about ten years ago, which sought to draw young people into a bawdy weekend of drinking, eating and love-making by calling to mind the ancient tradition of honouring May as the month of the fire gods.

On the way up the hill on a Friday evening there was a young man ahead of me, wearing sandals and a cloak. He had a fake hatchet and sword strapped to his back. His companion looked like an Apache in a blanket. Three boys from Ratharney were drinking from cans of Druids cider as a Garda helicopter circled the hill.

Four horses passed, their riders cloaked in maroon blankets, their faces painted black.

At the top of the hill there was a vast saucer-shaped meadow, more than forty acres, which was dotted with wicker huts, wigwams and sculptures of horses and other creatures, made from willow rods. There were stalls selling cider and roasted pig, potato cakes and rashers. There was a vegetarian soup, a bouncy castle and hundreds of people eating sausages, and listening to Sharon Shannon playing her concertina.

A motorised glider with blue wings crossed the sky. There was a tent for tattoos and a crannóg on stilts in a pond, and children were running everywhere.

Everyone was unwinding. Phoning each other. Eating bacon. Looking for music sessions. There were ribbons on a hawthorn bush in the middle of a clump of stones.

At 9.30 p.m. the crowd gathered on the highest point of the hill, around a pile of wood that reached thirty feet into the sky, and the main ritual began.

The red sun was just setting as a procession of fire-dancers with flaming torches, lanterns and masks came up the slope, fire-throwers and drummers leading the way.

It was nothing like the tame street parades at arts festivals that I had been familiar with, where children dressed up as exotic fish, or dragons from China.

This was wild. And it felt both curiously indigenous in a Celtic way, and pagan.

The darkness deepened. The fire-dancers approached the top of the hill.

In terms of Greek drama this was the enactment of conflict between Darkness and Light played out before our eyes, with all the shamanic force that allowed the observers feel in their hearts the same drama as was happening before their eyes.

Impending darkness, the invisible antagonist, haunted the sky, and threatened rain, and gradually enveloped the earth.

But the protagonist was flame, a source of hope.

The ordinary folk on the hill were a witnessing chorus. And I felt I was remembering something other than the dull orthodoxy of Christian history. I was reaching back beyond Corpus Christi days, or Lady Days, patterns or pilgrimages, or Bilberry Sundays, to recover a more ancient memory from the collective unconscious.

I was standing in some wild night fifteen hundred years ago when fires were lit on the same hill to herald in the summer season, and to invoke good fortune, good crops and a good harvest.

When the enormous stack of wood ignited, the crowd cheered, and the young people found places to sit down – enchanted, in love or just dazed by the magic of the leaping flames.

Summer had come. It had been inaugurated by proper ritual.

People sat around the fire as if some fragment of eternity had broken through the night, for everyone.

Teenagers wrapped in blankets gazed at each other, full of desire, as if they had stepped not just into summer, but through a portal to some magical 'now' where they were about to enjoy the time of their lives.

I walked back down the path, where angels sculpted from papier-mâché stood in line with outstretched wings. I passed a boy and girl hugging each other at an upturned barrel of flames, their faces lit like something from Caravaggio's dreams.

As I got into my jeep at the foot of the hill I could hear the screech of the uileann pipes above tearing the darkness asunder, and far above me a paper lantern holding a tiny flickering flame floated in the night sky.

The far away hornpipe

The summer of 2018 was dry and warm. I spent days gazing at the lake. And I wondered if prayer and re- ligious devotion is easier to swallow in good weather. The ripe fields, the tossed hay, the yellow flowers and the sound of birds in the trees open the heart.

The rational mind slips down into the heart, and opens to the landscape as a child might open on its mother's lap. Faith is a childlike thing. But then so is love, and poetry.

I suppose the ancient monks were children and heart surgeons, tai chi masters of the western world. Healing internal wounds, and laying waste the destructive demons of the psyche. Technicians of compassion. Calm abiders. Observers of nature. Students of the fish. And musicians. Composers of poetry and singers of matins, vespers and other songs that channelled the energy of the cosmos in all its mysterious transcendence into the phrases of a simple poem.

And it's hard to imagine them during Leitrim's wet winters. But like my mother, they are just beyond my fingertips. And on warm summer days, I can see them in the fields.

I sat in my studio with an icon of the Great Mother. And even though I woke at night with pains in my hip and choking for breath like a drowning man, the weather tried to reassure me that the universe meant well.

When I tried a short walk up the hill, my muscles creaked, like they had lost their elasticity, and I would abandon the walk and tell myself that I was old.

194   I would sit on a chair outside my studio, or on the patio, admiring the trees.

Sometimes I felt unusually cold and I sat by the stove, my cheeks going red as I poisoned myself in an airless room.

The beloved would appear at the door and say, 'It's very stuffy in here.'

The more I closed myself off in the studio, the more a distance began to grow between us.

'Perhaps we need a holiday,' she suggested, one day in the beginning of July.

Over the years we grew to understand that people can become lost in the mundane, and a couple can lose each other in the ordinary things of life. Sharing a house, a family, two careers and a cat can become routine. It all runs like a clock. And a week away is always refreshing.

'What about Tenerife,' I wondered.

She agreed. We went. And I got seriously sunburned on the

first day. After that I kept indoors or in the shaded corridors of shopping malls staring at inane souvenirs, and drinking cool beers and eating pizzas.

The plane journey took so long that I began to realise that Tenerife was geographically part of Africa, though politically it might be part of Spain. I would look out to sea at leisure boats, ski boats and the gliders floating in the air behind the speedboats on the azure ocean, and I'd wonder what might happen if a boatload of refugees ever darkened the horizon. What reception might they get from the north European holidaymakers, with red flaking sunburned skin falling off their arms, as they bought leather handbags in the tented city of stalls along the waterfront or tablecloths from the Senegalese men who kept moving through the sand, with the brightly coloured cloth draped like sashes across their shoulders.

Tenerife was not our home. Neither of us enjoyed sun holidays. They were boring.

Why were we there, on the beach, gluttonous for more drink and food every day, and lounging half-naked on a sunbed while groups of African men squatted in shaded corners and talked about how to get a few euros from the tourists.

Two days after returning from Tenerife I went to the doctor for a check-up. I didn't tell him I was feeling low. I went through the blood pressure test like a boy hoping to get through an examination. He said I should watch my stress levels.

'Take it easy. You've been travelling a lot.'

195

I said, 'I'm going to Warsaw next week.'

And it was true. I had booked the flight when we were booking for Tenerife.

So the betrayal continued, month after month, as I dived deeper and deeper into the solitary life and religious devotion.

'I'm a writer,' I said. 'I need to finish the book.'

The beloved was silent. She's a sculptor. We're both artists. The autonomy of our work is an uncontested territory. If I said I needed to go to the moon to write a book she would not object.

196   That gave me a certain licence.

I knew that I wouldn't finish any book now, and I wasn't going for that reason. The writing was over. The betrayal had deepened. This had nothing to do with the beloved. I was betraying myself.

I was in Warsaw once again on the final week of July, just seven days after we returned from Tenerife.

The baby in the pram

I often sit in Giovanni's restaurant in Carrick-on-Shannon – a traditional, old-style chip shop, with gleaming tables and tiled floors, where the chips are always fresh and the Diavola pizza is a work of art. But most of all I like it because it's anonymous. I'd often sit there for ages, during bad weather with cups of tea, watching the light on the street outside come and go as the snow fell and stopped and fell again.

One day a young man with a long scraggy beard came in and sat beside me. I was alarmed because clearly he was determined to interrogate me.

'Are you a pram baby?' he inquired.

I wasn't sure what he meant.

'In my lifetime,' he confided, 'a lot of men who were confined to prams for long periods never got over it. And I seen you on *The Tommy Tiernan Show* recently talking about religion and I says to myself, there we go again, Patsy, another pram baby!'

'Patsy,' I said, presuming it was his name, 'are you having something to eat?' as the waitress came with my plate of chips and beans.

I hoped the question might encourage him to go away. But it didn't.

'Thanks,' he said, without shame, 'I'll have a mug of tea.' My strategy had backfired.

'All that old shite about religion and God that you and Tiernan go on about,' he declared, 'that's all pram-baby talk.'

His beard and hair were dirty. I presumed he didn't have running water in whatever galvanised cottage he sheltered in on the side of some Leitrim mountain.

'The compulsion to write goes back to the pram,' he explained. 'The afflictions of the storyteller are nurtured in childhood loneliness. You sit alone all day putting words on a page. But its torture. And the only reason you do it is because you were stuck in a pram at an early age, and isolated from the world so severely that you began inventing things: like God. Am I right or wrong? And then after the God period, you start into other stories. Am I right or wrong?'

In fact I do remember the pram, and being pushed into the garden when I was an infant for such long periods of time that I ended up thinking I was a tree. And I was so lonely out there that I longed for other humans and when I heard distant voices, I thought they came from heaven.

When I was ten years old I heard a Christian Brother say that saints were special because they heard voices.

'But, brother,' says I, 'I hear voices all the time. Isn't that why we have ears?'

'Don't be smart-alecky with me, ye pup ye,' the brother replied, and he opened the palm of his hand and slapped me on the cheek so intimately that I could smell his aftershave.

'Do you come in here often?' the young man with the long beard asked as I ate my chips.

'Do you write every day?' he inquired.

'How well do you know Tommy Tiernan?' he wondered.

'Do you suffer with the nerves?'

By the time I had finished the chips and beans he had stripped me of all privacy. And yet I liked him.

His face quivered with a terror that comes from being swallowed by a forest of spruce trees, and from too many years in a damp cottage, with too little money and too much marijuana and no television licence, perhaps. His hands weren't washed and his fingernails were chafed.

'Were you left in a pram too?' I wondered.

'Don't talk to me about it,' he said, wincing at the memory.

'So why come to Leitrim?' I asked.

'Humans can't change much,' he said, with resignation. 'The pram defines everything. I learned to live with loneliness. And when I grew up what else could I do but continue in the same manner. In a pram. Or a forest. In me own head. Talking to nobody and wondering where has mother gone.'

'What do you do?' I inquired.

'I'm a poet,' he said, as defiantly as if he was telling me that he ate babies for his dinner.

And when he was gone there remained no doubt in my mind that writing has indeed everything to do with loneliness. And that sometimes poetry gets born in the darkest corner of the forest.

200

Accidental events

The first typewriter I owned was a gift from Uncle Oliver, my mother's brother, and a man of simple pleasures. A bachelor who lived in a semi-detached house in Dublin and enjoyed orange juice and mint ice cream on summer days, and wore sandals even when he was cycling around the Phoenix Park, and relished cream on his apple tart with the enthusiasm of a deprived child. 'Shall we have apple tart with some cream,' he would ask, 'or will we have cream with some apple tart?'

Uncle Oliver could get you anything. There wasn't an aunt who didn't have some story about how he had helped fill in a crucial form for her, to get a pension or some state benefit or grant for home heating, or even sometimes discreetly given them the price of a new washing machine. So before I turned fifteen, and had already written two poems, published in the *Junior Digest*, and delivered a further poem to a children's programme on Radio Éireann, I asked him one day if he knew how I could get a typewriter.

'I'll find out,' he said, which gave me enormous hope.

In summertime we usually stayed with Uncle Oliver for a week in July, swimming every day in Portmarnock, where I was once bitten on the foot by a jellyfish. My mother would drive us to the beach where we would idle in the sand, with small buckets, or take an occasional dip in the waves, as my mother did knitting, or read *Woman's Own* for a few hours as she sat on a tartan Foxford rug.

The jellyfish was a drama of enormous proportions for both me and my mother, and that evening as I sat with my foot up on the sofa in the front room of his house on Croagh Patrick Road, he said he had a surprise for me. He invited me into the little dining room at the back, which he used as an office, because we always dined in the tiny kitchen, and there on his desk, among the cuttings from newspapers, the folders of civil service papers connected with his job and the chess pieces standing at attack in mid-game, was a square black box.

I didn't know what I was supposed to be looking at. I loved dearly this room of chess pieces, the polished furniture, the scattered notebooks of Irish words which my uncle gathered in Connemara in summertime when he walked from house to house in sandals, and the music sheets that he studied with relish and practised on the upright piano that stood in the corner of the room which we were warned never to touch in case it went out of tune. I loved the smell of everything and the wonder of its privacy and miniature grandeur.

202

Oliver indicated that the black box on the table was the object he wanted me to examine. There was a leather strap handle on one side, with a small button, or clip, well rusted, which he suggested I flick to open. I did so, and raised what turned out to be a lid, revealing the shining black body of the typewriter inside. I was almost as shocked as if I had seen a rabbit. And I gushed with confused joy, and my uncle calmed me down and showed me how to roll a sheet of paper through the back of the barrel, and then how to press the keys, the various letters, until my name appeared in print on the paper. He then handed me a sheet and invited me to do the same. To roll it into the back of the barrel, and to begin my life as a writer.

203

'If you learn the correct way to type then you could be like the girls in my office,' he said, 'who can do ten pages while they are looking out the window, and having a conversation about the weather.'

There was nothing in life more important than telling stories and being a writer. That's what I was born to be, and it's how I lived, until I was sixty-five, but in the summer of 2018 I felt it was over. In March I had taken a break from my weekly column in *The Irish Times* and though it was now July, I had no intention of returning to it. There was no reason. It was just over.

I didn't go back to Warsaw to write. I went back to sit in a church and do nothing. Be silent. Be like a monk who closes his mouth and sits in the dark and remains there until the demons rise up.

And then confront them.

Banish them.

Wait until they dissolve. And eventually, this monk will find in his silence the embrace, the kiss that is mystical.

Well, it sounds great. But it's a long shot. It's an elusive bird in the bush for which I was betraying myself.

Because a writer needs to be alone only for so long as it takes to get the story. Either alone or by listening in silence, the writer takes the story down and then returns it to the audience. The story must be told.

204   I had learned storytelling from two sources: from country people and from Travellers. It was a simple apprenticeship. I just listened.

In the houses of single men in west Cavan, or in the trailers of Traveller women in Tullamore, or in the family kitchens of elderly couples on the Leitrim hills.

Lovely men and women that are long dead and gone, though I still remember the simplicity with which they could sum up their entire life in a few sentences. Often I listen back to their voices, recorded in ghostly kitchens that were long ago tossed and covered with sitka forest.

In the old days country people were slow to talk about personal or emotional matters, so I couldn't ask them the kind of questions that anthropologists or journalists might ask.

Instead we chatted about weather or cures or the location of some nearby holy well.

Eventually an accidental phrase might trigger some acute

memory and then the meaning of an entire life would spill out in a torrent of words.

Every story contained an attempt to resolve the mystery of life, because meaning matters to a storyteller more than happiness.

One day I was talking to a man about his schooldays.

'I was no scholar,' he said. 'The teacher had hands like shovels and he'd put my head through the desk sometimes with a blow.'

He folded his arms, leaned back on his chair and held his head up, like he was giving evidence.

205

'The master would sit up near the fire, and we'd be standing around him,' he said. 'If you made a slip in your reading he'd jump like a greyhound and bate you down to the end of the room.'

I asked him if he was happy as a child. But rather than tackle that curiosity with further psychobabble he continued with his autobiography.

'Me father had a heart problem. He died at forty years of age. He was the boss man in the county home and he had a little office to sign people in, and it was down to him if a person got in or not. And he had a free house that came with the job. When he married they had eight children, but on the day he died, a nun came up and locked the gates to the house and told me mother she had to be out before she even buried him.'

Without help from me he had found a seam to the heart of his story.

'So me mother was a midwife and she had a pony and cart, and she delivered thousands of babies in her lifetime,' he declared.

Sometimes people's stories are animated by long-buried rage or anger about things that happened years ago, and I'd be obliged to lighten the conversation by making tea.

Nowadays people don't realise that the art of tea-making, and elaborate discussions about various blends of tea, were not just inane murmurings: they were a complex form of punctuation during emotionally difficult narratives.

206   'I remember a Traveller man coming to the house on his bike,' he continued, 'in the middle of the night, and me mother had to go off in the dark to the camp with her pony and trap and the man's bicycle in the rear of the trap. But that was an emergency. Mostly the Travellers used to camp down the road close to us, 'cos they knew she was there in the house.'

Finally he had arrived at the heart of his narrative.

'I was sowing spuds with her one day, and the guard came to take me back to school. It was lunchtime. So I went back and then the master came in his car, and drove up to the wall of the school as he always did after his dinner. I could see him from the classroom, hopping out of the car with the *Irish Independent* under his arm. But as he was coming in the front door I was going out the back door. And when the guard came looking for me again, I stood me ground.'

'And did you not go back again?' I wondered.

'Never,' he said. 'I told the guard I couldn't go to school 'cos I was too busy moulding spuds for me mother. And me mother agreed with me. And the guard was sent away.'

The kitchen darkened and it began raining.

'She was a great woman,' he whispered, with wet eyes, and he wiped his cheeks with the back of his hand and I guessed that it might be time to make the tea.

By the summer of 2018 I had betrayed that precious story-telling. Because I didn't go back to Warsaw with any further interest in a book. I went back to closet myself in the mysteries of theology, and wrap myself in the blankets of old-fashioned religious zealotry.

Walking through Dublin airport in late July towards the Ryanair desks at the far end of the terminal felt like a final move. Perhaps in some respects I would never be back.

Both the writer and the monk engage with solitude. But the writer always surfaces again, to tell the tale. The monk, on the other hand, may be annihilated in the dark, if he is successful in the great romance with God.

And if he is not successful, his soul may burn in a hell of self-imposed parody.

Spiritual writers are few and far between: Thomas Merton, Meister Eckhart or all the great mystics of the first millennium of the Christian Era, in the deserts of Egypt, whose work constitutes the great Philokalia of the Orthodox tradition. They all speak about annihilation of the soul, and

207

the darkness of God, with a seductive style, as if the very emptiness of the universe was the breath of God, the very presence of a transcendent Other.

But perhaps all they ever found was emptiness and sterility. And despondency.

And renouncing the world is not something you can undo; as Irish mammies used to say about imperfect marriages, you made your bed, you must lie in it.

So it is with renunciation; if you turn your back on the world it's hard to climb out of the hole.

208   Up until recently, Coptic monks had no burial service, because it was understood that when they took their robes and entered on the path of solitude they were already dead. They had already gone away.

That should have frightened me. I had a partner to whom I ought to be faithful, not an abbot.

But by the time I got on the plane again in late July, I felt there was no turning back from the alluring wonders of any old icon.

And I fancied that I could be a tourist in the Cloud of Unknowing without getting burned any more severely than if I had lain out all day under the noonday sun in Tenerife.

This time I found an apartment by the river, on Bujaj Street, close to the Media Park where everyone gathered on Friday evenings to eat pierogis, burgers and ice cream and listen to pop music or classical favourites and allow their children put on swimming togs and run through the fountains.

Each day was filled with sunlight and clean white clothes and dazzlingly clean children. The cobbled stones of Old Town were polished by the leather of a thousand boots as tourists sprawled around the streets that six months earlier had been empty apart from me.

I sat at a table on the street and tried to see beneath the surface. I saw the past inside the present. I remembered the frost, the snow, the cold air blooming before my mouth like clouds. The muffled women with fogged-up spectacles gingerly edging their way along these same cobbled streets for something. And in the churches I felt the ghosts of people long dead, just beyond my fingertips.

I had no peace now other than with my icons in the shaded churches. And the shadows in those churches became exquisitely comfortable in summertime. Just as I had warmed myself in the cosy, heated interior of the Church of the Holy Cross in February, so now in July I went in to get away from the heat. I'd sit with my pants full of sweat, and beads of perspiration dripping down inside my shirt, and from my armpits and forehead. But there in the cool silence I felt loved, embraced and safe.

I cannot say why I ever darkened the door of a church as a young man, or what accidental mixture of iconography and incense aroused me so much that I wanted to be ordained a priest.

There had been much political turmoil. The church had been renewed in the documents of the Vatican Council and was opening the windows and doors to modern ideas, opting for the poor so dramatically that I imagined myself as priest and poet, among the poor, with a companion at my side in some new liberated church of the future. But all that was upended by the Polish pope and I felt like I had hopped on the wrong bus and needed to get off fast before it reversed completely into the nineteenth century.

So I did.

But I had also found a mother in the church; because I had missed the gestures of tender affection that one should associate with a normal childhood. So even from twelve years of age I thought that in the icons of the church I could find and be enveloped by all the tenderness that I had already missed.

Now that I'm sixty-five I know life is just one accidental event after another. And one failure after another. That's all. When we impose a pattern on our lives, it's like putting a string through beads. We could leave all the beads on the floor and say they had no shape or meaning.

But I opt for pattern. It's a choice. And it's the same little beads and the same little events that make up a life no matter which way you look at it. Going to Warsaw in winter, or again in summer, were both accidents.

August 2018 was one more bead on the necklace of time.

How many days in that sunny month did I sit on the wooden bench at the back of some church, sweating, imbibing the perfume of solitary women, their heads bowed under scarves as they prayed with clasped fingers and joined hands, after telling their secrets to some stranger in a cassock who shifted about behind a curtain in the corner of the transept? I cannot count them all.

In February nobody laughed or idled about the streets, never mind the park benches. It was too cold.

Now they kissed everywhere. Women in bridal gowns, and men in dickie bows; they kissed standing up on park benches, in front of statues and on the stone plinth around the fountains. Young couples stretched on the grass, in restaurants and on the streets; everyone laughed together until long after 9 p.m.

211

It was only a short walk from the apartment by the river up the hill to Freta Street. A social street of diners by night. A long line of restaurants on summer evenings, humming by candlelight. The smell of steak and oregano, pizza and perfume in the air after dark. And then, at ten each night, everything closed. Street silence.

The Media Park might be in full flight with neon lights, and speakers pounding out hip-hop music as late as 9.55 p.m., but at the stroke of ten everything was unplugged. And the crowds vanished into thin air. And the streets were empty until the morning.

I loved mornings. The tables empty. The waiters and waitresses brushing last night's crumbs off the tables. The wine-stained tablecloths being bundled for the laundry van. New tablemats being placed. The sun promising another blistering hot day under blue skies. The world waiting for the young to come again and fall in love.

I sat at a white tablecloth one morning, under a white canopy, waiting for a waitress.

She came and went and left me with a long cardboard menu for breakfast. But it didn't interest me.

'I just want a big coffee and a croissant,' I said.

'We are just baking the croissants now,' she replied. 'It will take five minutes.'

Five more minutes extra in the world, I thought. Can it get any better?

The croissant arrived, and a mug of hot coffee with two handles, and warm milk in a glass jar. The croissant warm to the touch and moist inside, a cavern of soft buttery pastry.

Beneath the blue sky only a few people moved on the street. Young men in their thirties with fierce muscles and tattooed arms, leading little dogs that smiled at everything; puppies clearly happy to be out and about. Older men clearing their throats as if they had been drinking late into the night and smoking too many cigarettes, their eyes bloodshot and their skin as rough as an elephant's arse.

In the distance the first bell, from a church further down, calling people to mass. Already a few old women with headscarves and prayerbooks waddling along the footpath.

The waitress spoke in halting English and smiled at me. I smiled back and wondered what she would think of me, if she knew I was praying like a lunatic. If she knew that soon

I would be with the old women in the back of a church somewhere, offering prayers like smoke to an implacable God I no longer believed in.

One morning on Freta Street a man sat at another table. His red hair was oiled and parted at the side. He wore a white shirt and long black trousers. He was on the phone as he leafed through what looked like receipts. I guessed he was the manager, or some kind of accountant associated with the restaurant.

Then a young couple arrived. A boy and girl with the shock of sexual intimacy still resonating from their amazed faces.

213

They tested the chairs. Each time they tried to sit, the chair was too close to the table and seemed stuck, because the legs of the chairs were neatly folded into the legs of the table. I had the same difficulty when I arrived. It took a slight effort to lift the table with one hand, and drag the chair out. But they couldn't seem to figure it out.

The boy was tall, with black hair and short trousers. The girl's skin seemed luminous and hairless apart from the light folds of brown falling either side of her cheeks. I guessed they were Spanish. They had white shirts. They spoke Spanish. They were both tattooed on their legs and arms, but the linen they wore was stiff and clean. And because they couldn't manage the chairs I went over, and showed them how to pull each chair from the table.

'They leave them like that overnight,' I said, in English, as if I knew anything about the chairs.

And they didn't speak English, but they smiled in gestures of appreciation. I returned to the dregs of my coffee and they continued to fumble with the chairs but they still couldn't figure out how to separate them.

Eventually they opted for the curious intimacy of sitting hip to hip on a single chair. It barely sustained them. But they did it nonetheless, their bodies pressed up against each other, like they already missed the intimacy of a wild night and wanted nothing more than to be joined to each other physically for the rest of the day.

214   Sometimes I sat in the heat. Sometimes in the shaded trees of Saski Park. Sometimes in the room with the curtain on the balcony drawn across. I sat at the same table every morning, ate a little croissant and drank a bowl of coffee, like a priest at his altar. And the couples around me became a congregation.

Dreaming of clocks

One morning I went into a café and ordered black tea and scrambled eggs. The tea arrived in a glass beaker, and the eggs were soft and the three pieces of toasted bread were made of rye and barley.

I relished every morsel while fighting off a small fly who thought he might go for a paddle in the soft egg.

I ate with one hand, while the other was constantly on the lookout for him.

I drained two small cups of tea. I poured the last load from the pot into the cup and sat back to savour it. A slim young man with a shaven head and wearing an apron took away the plate. And just as I was about to crown the breakfast with the final cup of tea the fly landed on the rim; near the handle, where I would put my lips in a moment, to drink.

I could have pummelled him. Or squashed the living daylights out of him.

But there was something about holding back from attacking even a fly that exemplified non-violence and made me want to laugh. In fact the more angry I got with his tiny life the more ridiculous I felt.

But on that same morning I remember looking at my legs in the mirror and noticing that my muscles were fading away. And the pain in my arm had intensified. And a strange black gauze was coming over my field of vision. And my body closed down most afternoons so that I had no energy to go out in the evenings. Yet still I didn't realise how soft the heart was turning. The only thing I could see was my belly in the mirror and it sagged alarmingly. And shame crept up on me every day as the body withered.

A drooping face in the mirror showed no trace of the joy I imagined was filling my heart when I sat in empty churches. Despair embedded in my facial features was the only fruit of all those hours reaching upwards in prayer.

Nor was I aware of how quietly the heart pumps, right up until the last moment. Or of how hard it struggles with clogged arteries. How desperately it tries and fails to get fresh oxygenated blood down the limbs, the arms and legs or into the brain in sufficient quantity.

I couldn't care less about flies or puffins, or the children of Warsaw. All I dreamed of in those moments of despair before the mirror was the comfort of food.

I suppose that's the core of old age. When there is only food left, as consolation, but you can't even eat it.

I brought my flute to Warsaw and brought it home again without playing more than a few notes. It sat in a wooden case that once held Packie Duignan's flute, and which Packie gave to a friend when he was dying and who later passed it on to me. But it sat too long in the case.

One morning before the heat tightened the muscles around my lungs, I lifted it out, and assembled its three parts and blew into it as tears came to my eyes.

I had missed it so much. It was as if my heart needed the sound of it. I played a polka: 'The Dark-Haired Girl'. A John McKenna tune. I felt the music like sculpture in the vibrating air. And the silence between the notes astonished me. Winded me. And gave me a sore neck. And so I put it down and went for breakfast.

217

'You ought to have practised more on the flute,' the fly said later, as he sat on the lip of my tea cup. 'There was no need to start crying; you are a man smothered in melancholy.'

'True,' I agreed. 'Like a pebble in the oyster around which the pearl is woven, I am wrapped around my own pain. I am like the notes enfolding a great silence.'

'You're a right fucking poet,' the fly said.

'Fuck off,' I replied, flicking him away.

I usually returned to the apartment by noon so as to rest from the heat of the day on my bed. In the corner of the room there were two old cinema seats, joined together, as they would have been long ago in some pre-war movie theatre.

They were made of dark wood with soft burgundy upholstery. And for hours I sat with my back to the wall, sometimes imagining myself in a cinema, or in a monastic cell, hundreds of years ago, listening to the same city sounds outside the window.

The wind in the trees.

The laughter of children.

At night, when the Media Park closed, I sat until the moon was high, gazing at the bed where I slept and trying to imagine if I was real at all or just my own delusion.

The beloved was far away in Ireland, dreaming her own life.

But even still, sometimes she was with me, on the bed, listening to me as I talked my head off in whispers.

Other times, when I returned from a long walk I would sit on the balcony for no purpose other than to undo my sandals and throw off my shirt which was usually dripping with sweat.

I walked for hours at night during August. On my return I would stare at the bed and the two cinema seats feeling that there was something I was missing. Something I had not been paying attention to. Something in the room about to strike. But I couldn't figure out what it was.

When I was asleep I dreamed of clocks. When I was in bars I noticed clocks and remembered the dreams. When I was in restaurants I worked on my laptop and stared at the clocks and thought about a fifth-century monk in the deserts of Palestine, who wrote about despondency. Sometimes at the tram stop I'd fall into a daydream and the tram would pass, and leave me behind.

Solitude kicks in.

Even my phone went silent. As if people knew not to call.

Eventually I plugged it out and didn't recharge it. Nobody could contact me now. If I saw an email on the laptop I deleted it. Because it had no relevance.

I was gone to the cave, sometimes like a monk in communion with heaven, and sometimes like a vigilant bear who knows there is something out there in the dark.

Accidents in
the afternoon

And things didn't improve when I returned to Leitrim at the end of August. I had whipped up such a fer- vour for icons and prayers and delph statues in the shadows of old churches that I was determined to maintain a sort of spiritual retreat even at home.

When I got back, the beloved looked at me and said, 'You're tired.'

'No, I had a great time,' I replied cheerfully. 'It was like a retreat. Absolutely wonderful. Orthodox Christianity is fascinating. I'm reading a lot of books. The icons are talking to me.'

'Well,' she said, 'you look tired.'

That was the extent of the fracture.

All the plants on the patio had burned up that summer and even in August we could still sit out and barbecue steak and drink Bordeaux wine.

When I closed the door of my studio, and touched an icon, and ran my fingers along its surface, the gesture felt like an external shadow of what was happening inside me. I was reaching inwardly, towards the hidden core of my own self.

I longed to be awake; free from anxiety and at peace with the mythic gods of my psyche. And when I found the gods of my psyche made manifest in icons, the ego dissolved in a great surge of devotion.

Icons allowed me to surface in the present. I was beginning to understand their function.

On the patio one evening in late August the General was sitting by the barbecue and I tried to explain this to him.

222

'But are you writing anything?' he inquired, from under bushy eyebrows.

'I'm trying to finish a new book,' I lied, 'but I keep falling asleep. I go to my desk after lunch and I'm like a cat on the sofa.'

'It's the salad,' he suggested. 'You might be eating too many lettuce leaves.'

The General was convinced that anything green was always dangerous, even on the dinner table.

'We are beasts,' he declared, his eyebrows floating up his forehead.

'When we sit down to eat we need to make sure that there's blood running out of whatever is on the plate.'

He'd be even happier if he saw the flesh moving on the plate. But he considers lettuce to be particularly dangerous.

'Especially if you're driving a car,' he added. 'A lot of accidents happen in the afternoon. People don't drink at lunch but they stuff themselves with these salads from bowls as big as wash-hand basins. Then they get into a car and they're nodding off at the first traffic lights.'

'What on earth were you doing in Warsaw?' someone asked in the supermarket. 'You didn't need to go over there for good weather.'

'I was writing,' I lied again.

'Did you finish anything?'

'No.'

'You don't know what you want. No amount of nostalgia in the churches of Poland will help you write another poem.'

'True,' I said. The beloved was watching me. But she said nothing. She must have known all along that there was no book.

I worried that I might be standing where the great Donegal writer Seosamh Mac Grianna once stood when his well went dry and the writing was over.

He became so despondent that when the priest arrived with Holy Communion every Sunday morning in Letterkenny psychiatric hospital and offered the sacred host to Mac Grianna, he would just turn and say, 'Fuck off.'

Grief poured out

At the beginning of September I drove to Clare for the funeral of a young man, a carpenter who had met a sudden death. His mother was a poet. His friends were from a community of new-age, long-haired romantics the likes of which pepper the mountainsides of Ireland, west of the Shannon.

He was a beautiful boy, and in the tiny wake room of the funeral home people laid flowers, and a Buddha statue and a letter, at the foot of the coffin. In their grief, in their mellow tin whistle slow-air serenity, I could hear a keening like ancient Gaels as the coffin was closed. I cried to think of how unbearable the moment was for his mother and sisters and lover. And for his friends.

It seemed he had so many, all gathered about in the tiny room, around the coffin, and twice as many out on the street looking in the windows.

An old German man who had apprenticed the young boy spoke.

'We worked together for sixteen years,' he said. 'He was my life. For all those years, he was almost the only thing in my life.'

Outside, men with red faces and beards as long as the beards of mountain goats, and long cheap coats, smoked tobacco. They sported ponytails, and women stood in long dresses, wearing big earrings, so that it was clear to any of the passing Toyotas, clear to the middle classes going home from their mundane work and duties, that this was the burial of someone from an alternative culture.

And I felt the strength of their prayer. An eclectic, non-denominational murmur. And sometimes it felt like the weary sigh of new-age hippies, and sometimes it felt as ancient as the sorrow of monks a thousand years ago on the same rocky slopes of Ireland's west coast – a timeless cosmic prayer ascending to heaven, the dynamic of its grief renewing everyone who cried and wept.

When the poems had been recited, and the tobacco and whiskey smells dissolved, everyone travelled the road to the crematorium and all the time they prayed and sang.

Prayer is just a word for grief poured out. And I too was grieving for the lost year.

My heart was breaking. Waves of sorrow came like short breaths, and a longing to sit down every time I had to stand for more than twenty minutes.

I prayed.

Dear Christ, sorrowful wound in my psyche, and behind me, before me, above me, beside me, please help me.

I was grieving for a writer's life that was over. Or a bigger loss. I didn't quite know what train might be coming.

I was in my study one morning and there was a lovely stillness across the lake. I was listening to a CD of Rachmaninoff's Vespers which I got from a woman on the street in Clare the previous week.

She handed it to me without any reason. And when a woman comes out of the blue and points a man in a particular direction there is never a reason to argue. So I sat listening to the choir all morning and wishing I was alone in a monastery garden. To add my voice to the choir as they sang, 'Come let us worship.'

As a teenager I used to wonder why other young people were alienated from religion. What could be more wonderful, I thought, than the glow of fire in a bucket on Holy Saturday night?

I thought atheism was the cantankerous whim of grumpy students who happened to be more intelligent than me. I didn't realise that reading history had made them wise.

Although it wasn't the bombs falling on Dresden or the crooked smoke wafting from the chimneys of concentration camps that destroyed Ireland's enthusiasm for religion.

It wasn't even B-52 bombers showering napalm on Vietnam that marked the death of innocence in our hearts.

It was the unrelenting drip of stories about children raped and buggered by clerics that woke Ireland up. The grim and intimate narratives of child abuse had been the milestones in the nation's journey away from the pomp of Rome.

Yet in the autumn of 2018 I felt nostalgic for a long-ago time when I was eighteen years old and had stepped for the first time into religious life as a seminarian.

Back then my most treasured possession was a blue prayerbook containing the poetry of the psalms. I touched it and cared for it as if it were a living thing. As if it were a portal to another world. Each one of us carried a copy and we used it when we sang together at dawn or in the evenings. Twice a day we assembled in the oratory, in alphabetical order, so that a man's immediate neighbour in the pew never changed, and became a companion in prayer over years. A soul friend. And a way of building solidarity.

At night I reached out and touched the blue book of psalms on my bedside locker before falling asleep. I held it to my breast as I walked to the oratory on dark winter mornings across the snow-covered square past a life-sized crucifix that stood in the rosebeds – a cold, dead Christ in white marble with his arms outstretched. We thought the crucifix was a kind of compass, a hopeful sign in the snow. Although as I remember it now it was the rosehips that were beautiful in September, and it was the roses that have remained in my life as the sign of love.

Footsteps

On Saturday morning, 20 October, I got a phone call to say that Bernard Loughlin had died suddenly the previous evening after an accident near his home in the high Pyrennes.

For many years Bernard had been the director of the Tyrone Guthrie Centre, an artists' retreat in Monaghan. When I went there in 1984 I used to argue with him about religion. Not that I ever defended the ontological guff of metaphysics so popular with official churches, but I did contend that faith was a wholesome act of the imagination. Bernard argued robustly to the contrary. And we both relished our passionate disagreements.

On the day I heard of his death I took a flight to Barcelona, and drove up into the mountains of Catalonia. The following day I stood with a small crowd of friends as we watched the hearse zig-zag its way up through a valley and along a mountain path, on Bernard's last homecoming. Then everyone shouldered the coffin on the final few steps to his house, where his loved ones could touch for the last time his rugged face, and see his eyes closed forever, as they grieved for the man they loved so well.

I too loved Bernard. I loved him as a man sometimes loves another man; not as an equal or partner, but as a guide so close to one's own psyche that their accidental remarks seem to pave a way into the future. Such mentors have many names: guide, soul friend, elder. And they are valuable components in the fabric of any society, because impressionable young disciples swallow their charm, idolise their words and transform their ordinary mutterings into wise sayings.

Bernard Loughlin was erudite, well-travelled and widely experienced, so for me he was the perfect model of an elder, despite his passion for argument and controversy.

When I first encountered him in the garden of the Tyrone Guthrie Centre, I was terrified of him. He wore an old hat, and a tattered coat. He leaned on a digging fork, shuffling out young spuds.

'Just look at these, Monsignor,' he said, mocking me. 'Sure who would want heaven, when you can have a garden?'

When he wasn't in the garden, he policed the interior of the big house to ensure that slovenly artists did not disturb the ambience of quietude and ease that pervaded the space. He often chastised young males who didn't think that cleaning dishes was a manly task.

'You can take the boy out of the bedsit,' he would declare, 'but you can't take the bedsit out of the boy.'

He never minced his words, and he expected high standards from any artist who had been given the privilege of a residency.

I dreaded being caught putting plates in the wrong slots in the dishwasher. And even in the pub, I dreaded sitting next to him because he was so erudite I feared I'd be shown up as an illiterate gobshite.

Although I could recognise his footstep anywhere. Especially on the corridor that led to my room above the library. I had to jump off the bed frequently, and sit at the desk, so he'd think I was working on a novel.

231

But after all the years that have passed since then, I can say that nothing ever shaped me as a writer more than my first admission to the Tyrone Guthrie Centre, and Bernard's belief in me So as I stood in his mountain garden in the high Pyrennees, after the funeral, the suddenness of his death overwhelmed me. The tomatoes and peppers he plucked three days earlier still lay in a basket on the grass. A spade stood idle, against the ditch. And I wanted to say, 'Thank you, Bernard.'

But it was too late.

Begin again

Maybe it was those sudden deaths that gave me the urge to begin again, to find another house for me and the beloved. Somewhere to make our retirement years as precious as our first love.

I was sixty-five and another house would have been absurd. Even if we did have the money to buy one.

We had lived in the same house for twenty-five years. And we loved it. It was our paradise, surrounded by hardwood trees, a view of the majestic Lough Allen and Sliabh an Iarainn on the other side.

Why would we think of leaving?

It was another betrayal; first it was the beloved, and then myself as a writer, and now the very ground I stood on. The sacred space that held me together. Timpaun. The musical hill. The woodland that sheltered me.

All those trees, oaks and ash and beech. The glorious flowering of one hundred little saplings we had planted in 1994.

The little cottage rooms so full of cherished memories. The place where we stood; our ground. The sacred earth.

I would betray that too.

Although it began as a game.

The first house I looked at was in Portlaoise. It was near the filling station where I often stopped for lunch on my way down the country. And I was going down the country a lot during the autumn of 2018, touring with a new book.

Every night I'd read from the book, spending about ninety minutes on stage, and then I'd return to some hotel I had already checked into earlier in the afternoon.

And the following morning I would return to Leitrim.

Portlaoise happened to be a good halfway stop, and the filling station had a carvery counter that served fresh lunches.

The house wasn't far away; a semi-detached, with a C BER rating, three bedrooms and a lovely fireplace in the front room which was open to the dining area. And though there wasn't much room outside, I imagined myself sitting at the back of the house, which was south-facing, with a book and a glass of wine at the weekends. In this fantasy my beloved would be in a studio somewhere nearby, making art, and on the weekends we'd be up and down to Dublin on the train, which would cost nothing since by now we were both old-age pensioners.

This fantasy was founded on the fact that the property was on sale for a hundred and thirty-nine thousand euros, and our small cottage in the hills above Lough Allen could easily realise that kind of money. Or so I hoped.

It was a fantasy about beginning again. Of having a new life. And sometimes anywhere seemed attractive. The faraway hills are greener, but the notion that the faraway housing estate could even match the idyllic mountain retreat our home had become was absurd.

Maybe it's because there was nothing exciting on the television that autumn. Or maybe because I was bored with the rain in Leitrim after twenty-five years of it. Or maybe just because I was sleeping less and my mind seemed to have more space for idle daydreams.

Whatever the reason, I became committed to the search.   235

So I mentioned it to the beloved. At first she didn't think it was such a great idea.

I dropped the subject.

But the week wasn't over before she had taken a peek at other houses in other parts of the midlands to see if there was anything on offer that she thought interesting.

It was just a game. An alternative to Facebook. But I had her hooked.

'There's an interesting house for sale in Banagher,' she said. She was joking.

'We should look at it,' I said, 'just for fun.'

But it wasn't a game for me. So I searched the details and found a large empty premises on the main street, with dwelling quarters above the shop and a long garden of mature trees at the rear. It had the imposing austerity of an old convent, with thick walls and narrow slit-like windows.

And I saw that as a plus. A good sign. Anything remotely religious excited me. It was so enclosed from the street that it could easily be a place of silence and retreat for years.

'Yes,' I said, 'we should have a look at it.'

'Are you serious?' she asked.

'Yes. Well, maybe not. No,' I said, backing off. 'Actually not at all. No. No interest.'

And that was the end of that one.

'But there is a very good bargain in Ballinasloe,' I added.

That was the game. Keep sincerity out of it but see what came up. Just for a laugh.

'Well,' she said, 'I would always need a studio if we ever moved from Leitrim.'

'But would you ever move?' I wondered.

'I'd never say no to anything,' she replied.

'OK,' I said, 'that building in Banagher has a shopfront on the ground floor facing onto the street, so that could be converted.'

'It could,' she said. But we were bluffing each other. Propped up on pillows, with separate laptops, it was all a bit of fun. Daring each other to think outside the box.

I had started something. Now it was taking on a life of its own.

The hunt was on. The game continued.

'But I'm happy here,' she said, alarmed when she realised I was growing more serious. 'Why would we move?'

I had no answer.

I usually did gigs every Friday and Saturday, and the tour went on for two and a half months. I was in Sligo at the end of a week, and decided to drive home afterwards. I was tired of hotels.

The Sligo show went well. A full house. Lots of laughs.

In the dressing room I packed away my stage suit, shoes and the sound equipment, wheeled out my suitcase to the Skoda and put everything in the boot. Then I headed for home. It was an hour's drive, and when I arrived I settled down at the television, replayed a few news programmes, had a few glasses of wine and went to bed.

I woke in the morning beside the beloved and we talked houses again. It was a way of passing time in bed too.

The following week I was in Carlow and even there, I decided to return directly after the show even though it was a three-hour drive. I was at the television again, till after one o'clock, and I got excited with Brexit as it unfolded slowly on a news channel and I drank an entire bottle of wine on my own.

I was so sick the following day that I promised myself never to drink like that again. I guessed that the reason the wine floored me so dramatically was because I drove all the way home after the gig and I was tired.

So I switched back to the old system. Get a hotel and stay over after a show no matter where it was.

Two weeks later the beloved was in London and I was on stage in Dundalk. I had a hotel arranged. I booked in around 4 p.m., and I noticed a bottle of wine on the bedside locker, already open, with two wine glasses beside it.

Very strange.

But perhaps it was meant for someone else. Perhaps the staff confused the rooms.

I ought to have phoned reception and told them there was a bottle of wine in the room and it wasn't mine.

But I didn't.

Again I had a full house in the large town hall, and when I returned the bottle of dark Spanish Rioja was sitting exactly where it had been before I left.

So I decided to take a glass.

Just one.

And then I had another. Which was very pleasant.

And then another.

Until the bottle was empty and I began to imagine a dark angel, a tall spectre in the shadowed corner, standing beside the now empty bottle.

The room was full of shadow anyway because the little bedside lights never cast their light very far. And I grew more certain that I could feel a presence.

The following morning I was very sick. And I could hardly drive home.

Later in the day, I was forced to negotiate the winding roads of Monaghan, Armagh, Fermanagh and Cavan, weaving in and out of the UK a dozen times as I ranted about Brexit.

Eventually I reached Leitrim, still wondering where the bottle of wine had come from and determined never to take another drink until the tour was over.

There were twenty more gigs to go, through the autumn, from Kerry to Wexford, Galway, Mayo, Donegal and Kildare. And lots of dates in Dublin.

And I varied my strategy. Sometimes I booked a hotel and stayed over after a show no matter where it was. Sometimes I went home, had a mug of tea with a slice of apple tart, watched the latest report on Sky News about Brexit and went to bed.

Whenever I woke beside the beloved, at home, I was usually wired to the moon, full of unrelieved adrenalin and stories about who I had met at the show the night before.

239

While we sipped coffee and sat up on pillows, I explored the internet for more exotic places to live other than Leitrim. Searches which usually related to where I had been the night before.

If I was doing a gig at the Wexford Opera House I would search daft.ie and other property sites the following morning for places in Wexford.

'Why are we doing this?' she wondered.

'Because maybe Leitrim will be lonely,' I suggested, 'as we get old. Maybe a time will come when we won't be able to live on the side of a mountain, with a beautiful view, and we will regret we didn't move to a town.'

'That's a grim thought,' she said.

'I know,' I agreed.

And in October I crashed the Skoda into the arse of an old Volvo as I was returning from a gig in Dublin.

'You only ever crash the car when you are not physically well,' she observed.

I thought that was funny.

The following week the car was fixed. And I reversed it into a bush in the garden and had to get the back door replaced.

She said nothing.

Then I noticed a house for sale in Galway.

'Look,' I said to the beloved in the bed. 'It's close to a gym.'

But she wasn't for Galway.

'Although Cork could be interesting,' she countered. So we looked at Cork.

240

And Mullingar.

Kinnegad.

Dromad.

And finally Donegal.

The reasons for finding a house varied, from one week to the next, through an erratic autumn of touring, but the compulsion to grasp something, anything, was as constant as a drowning man's eye on a remote life raft.

By then we were no longer looking for a house in a town. Now we were searching for rural properties. It didn't matter that the original reason was to find a townhouse for our retirement.

We just did it like we might wander through Facebook, surf for new laptops, search for video reviews of cars or just read the newspapers online.

'What about a house by the sea?' she suggested.

'That's a great idea.'

I didn't question why we had not thought of such a plan twenty years earlier.

'I am only sixty-five,' I argued. 'In the prime of my life. Just the perfect time to move house and begin again.'

Every time a show was over, I went home, watched television, slept, woke and found another house.

It was the middle of November and it was time to begin the slow lead-in to Christmas.

And I saw the perfect house in Athlone. It was Sunday morning and I begged her to come and look at it.

She agreed, and we drove down to Athlone after breakfast. We peeked in the windows. We had a drink downtown with a friend from years ago who we met accidentally on the street.

I felt my grip tightening on this house. I needed it.

The following day I phoned the auctioneer and left a message on his answering machine. A few hours later she called back to say that the house was no longer available.

I was devastated.

But the following Sunday morning, after yet another gig, I was in bed and the beloved was on her laptop, and I was lying with my eyes closed reciting Orthodox prayers when she said, 'Just look at this lovely little holiday home in Glencolmcille. Have you seen it?'

It was a dainty cottage in the village, opposite the folk park and beside the beach, for sale at a reasonable price. Instantly I felt it was ours.

On Monday I phoned the auctioneer. I got intoxicated again with the idea. And we drove all the way to Glencolmcille and examined it that afternoon even though the light was almost gone from the sky when we arrived at the door and met the auctioneer.

But it was perfect.

No heating.

But that didn't matter.

The floors were coming up in spots. But that could be fixed. The guttering was broken. But it would be no bother to get someone to sort that out. And the view wasn't great. But it was in the valley. It was beside the beach. Sure for God's sake it was perfect. I was so excited that I got extremely short of breath.

The next day I made an offer. The owners accepted. I went crazy with delight. I wired a booking deposit to the auctioneer immediately.

'You might as well say it's ours,' I declared.

'In all my eighteen years working in this profession,' the auctioneer replied in an email, 'I don't think I've ever received a deposit so quickly. It goes without saying that we can't thank you enough.'

It was a feeling that the gods knew what we wanted. That the universe had spoken. That we had been guided. That our eyes had been directed all along through the weeks of looking towards this final end.

Some people's destiny was death.

Some to die suddenly and unexpectedly.

But ours was different.

Ours was to begin again.

And I was desperate about it; I needed to believe in it. My energy was just too low to think otherwise.

I couldn't sleep. I had a pain between my shoulder blades. It bored its way right through me to the front of my chest. I never called it chest pain. I never thought of it as chest pain. It was only a pain in my back. Probably came from sitting too long bent over the typewriter, I thought.

And whatever the cause of the sore back, the house was the answer. Whatever despondency, or physical ailments, or 243 general exhaustion from ageing that was oppressing me, they were all symptoms that would be dissipated instantly if we secured another house.

Another life.

This house was luck. Like the greatest thing that ever happened us.

Life is just beginning. We'll go and start a new life. Sure for God's sake we're only in our sixties.

There would have been no sane or rational reason to sell the beautiful home that we loved and that had sheltered us for a quarter of a century. No reason to fly off to the coast of Donegal in our mid-sixties to begin again, with all the horror of negotiating builders, and planting hedges, and fixing broken doors, and trying to connect with the community, just so we could live in a remote landscape. Especially since the beginning of the search was directed towards finding a house in a town where we wouldn't be isolated in old age.

It was completely insane. And yet I was driven to realise it. We tied ourselves to it even before we could begin to figure out how to raise money from our own home.

Would we sell it?

Yes, I thought, for sure; because there was one single reason why the house in Donegal was worth it.

And that reason was the name: Glencolmcille. The name was enough for me.

Glencolmcille is remote, and turns itself towards the Atlantic in spectacular fashion, with high cliffs and beautiful isolated beaches enveloping the parish. There are megalithic tombs, and standing stones used in ancient rituals of the pre-Christian era all across the valley. And at some stage in early Christian times it was renamed as the valley of Colmcille, and it was said that the monk spent two years there on retreat and wrestled with demons at the shoreline near the town of Kilcar.

But despite being shrouded in a cloak of superstition and folklore, Colmcille was indeed born near Letterkenny in the sixth century.

He was a monk. He established monasteries. On the island of Iona off the Scottish coast, he established a major centre, teaching his monks to read and write and copy manuscripts, developing links with other monasteries, and eventually dying there, one morning just before beginning the divine services for the day. He was seventy-five. They buried him on the island, though his relics were taken back to Ireland

244

two hundred years later, just before the Vikings arrived to plunder Iona, and they were interred with those of Patrick and Brigid in Downpatrick because by then he had become one of the three great apostles of Ireland.

All this is history, and would be of little relevance to me except that I had become convinced that the Irish Celtic church would have been much more in accord with the theology and practices of Orthodox Christianity than with the Roman tradition which came later.

It's no accident that the Trinitarian nature of God was the most central tenet of faith in the Celtic church and that Patrick was always associated with the shamrock for good reason. It's no accident that so much music and poetry can be linked back to the ancient chanting of monks, and it's no accident that the great books of Kells, and Durrow, and other places, were all steeped in the grammar of iconographic art that is today the mark of prayer in much of the Orthodox tradition.

I became convinced that Colmcille was a wise man, a writer, a monk, and that he would have been familiar with the theology and liturgies of Eastern Orthodoxy.

I had no scholarly evidence for this but I was beyond reason. I was living by signs.

That there was a house for sale on the west coast of Donegal was one fact. That I had been absorbed by the exotic colour of Orthodox ritual and theology for over a year was another fact.

All I needed was a sign to link the two. And Colmcille was

the man, the monk and the sign that brought it all together.

Magical thinking had unbalanced me.

The beloved had her own reasons for entering this whirlwind of imaginative adventure, although she never got around to airing them fully. But she was an artist who had always known that art is the tracks of the animal and that the life of an artist is essentially about taking risks on the basis of one's intuitions.

As Tom MacIntyre used to say regularly, when both of us were downing a few glasses of wine and discussing the nature of the writer's life, 'An artist must walk over the cliff, blindfolded.'

246

We could talk it over through Christmas. We could look at the positives and negatives, and see what we might get for our own home if we sold it, and since we had a booking deposit of three thousand euros paid, the house would be secure until at least January.

'But why commit so soon?' she asked. 'Should we not wait?'

'Oh no,' I said, 'we can't wait. What if someone else comes looking for it? What if something else happens? No, we must strike while the iron is hot.'

That was in late November. I could sense catastrophe around the corner. I sniffed it. But I couldn't put my finger on it. And then of course there was the great coincidence concerning the nuns.

THE SLOW AIRS
OF THE MOUNTAIN

Completing a miracle

The nuns who appeared in my life in the autumn of 2018 were like the completion of a miracle. Even though they were not in fact nuns, nevertheless they became the final piece of the jigsaw, convincing me that a hidden hand was directing my life like a play. From the moment the wine appeared on the bedside locker in the hotel in Dundalk, to the payment of the deposit on a house we didn't need, things were coming together. I could feel it in my body at night – and in the duvet, like it was made of lead and pressing down on my chest. Something strange was happening. How wonderful, I thought.

I remember being in a small town not far from Athlone one night, reading from my book in the local arts centre. Afterwards some of the audience queued in the foyer with books for me to sign.

After a few signings, a shy man wearing a tattered raincoat buttoned up to his neck stood before me like a stranded cow in a field of rushes.

'I have something for you.'

He took a tiny plastic statue of Padre Pio from his pocket. A small cream and brown figure, probably made in a factory beyond in Asia. It certainly wasn't a work of art. And it was clear from the saint's garish face that the makers didn't have much clue about mystical contemplation in the lives of Christian monks.

Padre Pio can be scary enough at the best of times, especially with holes in his hands, but this particular grinning monk was so garish that he resembled someone intending to chop up the cat into tiny pieces.

I accepted the gift with gratitude and went back to my hotel, where I disposed of it in the wastepaper bin.

But I couldn't sleep.

And I guessed it was because disposing of a saint in the dustbin was not a way to develop good sleep karma. So I took him out, and stood him on the dressing table and apologised. When I turned off the light I could feel him still looking at me, but I slept like a baby, and in the morning, as I opened my eyes, I wondered what to do with him.

It wasn't right to abandon him in a small hotel near Athlone. And I didn't want to take him home. So it was a difficult conundrum to solve, as I stood at the bedroom window, until I noticed a church across the street.

The perfect place to bid him farewell, I thought.

The morning mass was just over. A handful of elderly people were arming themselves with umbrellas inside the porch, ready to brace the sleet. And a tiny little woman was shuffling about the nave, turning off lights.

As I knelt in a pew and gathered my thoughts into a half-baked state of mindfulness, the old lady spoke in loud whispers to another elderly woman who was sitting a few benches behind me.

'I'm sorry, Mary,' the first woman said, 'but I must turn off the lights now. I hope you don't mind. Father Cardigan said we were to save money on electricity so I'm trying not to leave too many on after mass.'

To which the second woman replied, 'The only light we need in here is yourself. You brighten up the place for everyone.'

251

They both laughed, and then the first lady moved away and clicked another switch on the wall.

Outside the morning was frosty and a grey winter sleet battered the back door. Eventually the woman behind me genuflected, but instead of leaving, she came up to where I was sitting.

'I'm the last nun in this town,' she said proudly. 'I have a little apartment, off main street. The convent closed years ago.'

'The nuns disappeared very fast in the end,' I said.

'Like snow off a rope,' she agreed. 'But sure the same will happen the bishops in the next few years.'

She paused and then, rather brightly, added, 'I'm eighty-two, but I hope God spares me to see that.'

We chatted a while in the porch later, and I bade her farewell at the gates outside, and watched her frail body as she negotiated the slippery pavement and disappeared around the corner of main street. Padre Pio was still in my pocket, but I resolved to take him home and give him a prominent position among all the Buddhas on my Shelf of Holy Objects. And it was because the old woman had made such an impression on me with her anonymous serenity that I mentioned the other nuns to the beloved later that day when I returned home.

Three years earlier the beloved had met them in Warsaw, selling icons on the street. They'd come from a monastery in Minsk. The beloved was interested in the artistic aspect of icon-making, but she'd developed a camaraderie with the two nuns at the stall on the street, exchanging jokes, examining their wares and purchasing some of the soaps and ointments that they were selling, and eventually they'd exchanged emails.

They'd kept in touch and she'd invited them to come visit us in the hills above Lough Allen when they were in Ireland that winter.

They'd arrived in November, to sell their religious wares at church bazaars and Christmas markets from Dublin to Galway. They'd emailed first and then called to us one afternoon on their way to Sligo.

Two middle-aged women in white uniforms like nurses from the First World War. Their van driver was a lanky boy called Brother Dimitri, but he had no English and spent his time on the sofa bent devoutly over his smartphone.

The sisters had tea but refused food. They showed us inside the van, cluttered with icons, sanctuary lamps, hand-made soaps and ointments. I bought two icons of the mother of God, for ten euros each.

The sisters came into my studio to see the icon my beloved had made two years earlier in Warsaw. But my studio was bedecked not only with Christian icons of saints and angels and many Christs in various forms of agony and transformation, but also with numerous Buddhas, male and female, and Tibetan lamas hanging on the same walls.

The nuns appeared dizzy with this eclectic mix of deities. And they didn't linger. One sweeping glance, a quick examination of the Christian icons and they were gone. They fled back to the house, finished their mugs of tea and were away in the van with undignified haste. We had not heard from them since.

When I returned with Padre Pio in my pocket, and lodged him with the other holy saints, I suggested to the beloved that we should keep in touch with the nuns.

'It's probably my fault that they never came back,' I suggested, and she didn't disagree with me.

I went on their website and tried to purchase an album of choral chant. But I couldn't. My attempts returned an automatic reply saying that in order to purchase a CD I needed to email Sister Bernarda with my request.

So I did.

I presumed to hear back in a few days. But by coincidence a separate email arrived within an hour to the beloved, saying that two of the sisters were coming to Ireland soon, and wanted to pay her a visit.

The coincidence delighted me. Such signs, I thought. Such great omens.

And I wanted nuns in the house. Ever since those quiet hours I spent in the Orthodox cathedral in Warsaw I longed for the accoutrements of that faith, like a child might wish for gaudy trinkets. The idea of nuns under the roof was bliss.

254   Although they were not real nuns. Nuns would mean those black-robed women in elaborate headdress who could be seen on YouTube videos, singing, praying or gazing into the camera. Some of them looked like they might have been surreal painters in a former life. Some of them had the same lifeless severity in their gaze as the orphanage nuns of Ireland's disturbing past.

So I expected two middle-aged women in black drapes. But instead two young volunteers arrived, in white, whom I struggled not to speak of as girls, although that's how they appeared.

Two young lay sisters, in the same old-fashioned nurse outfits, going around Ireland in a van, selling icons. They were driven by the same lanky boy as before, who held the same phone as before and had not lost his enthusiasm for sitting on the couch playing internet games.

They arrived two days after I came home with Padre Pio.

They were beautiful, angelic, almost cinematic in their glowing sanctity.

I loved them and their red battered van, as it struggled up the hill like the travelling grocery shop that, years ago, traversed all of west Cavan. An old Bedford van, carrying provisions up lonely laneways on the slopes of Cuilce mountain, to elderly people who didn't get to town very often, or German hippies who had no car and lived in derelict cottages and reared their babies without disposable nappies, even though the travelling shop always had a few packets of Pampers hidden discreetly under the washing powders.

255

We weren't familiar with strangers back then. So we would weave a story around them. For example, people said that one of the German women on the mountain was so strong that she could carry bags of coal from Swanlinbar on her back. And according to gossip, there were Russian scientists working in the old Arigna power station, who had come from nuclear facilities in the Soviet Union. There was no end of stories that kept us warm in winter. But I never actually met the Russians, and I never saw any German woman walking with coal on her back. No more than I ever met Shergar in Ballinamore.

So maybe they were all just stories we told ourselves in the deep mid-winter, as a protection from despondency, or death in a cowshed. And maybe that's why I was glad when I saw the sisters come from Belarus. It's not just the holy icons that cheered me, or the fact that their van reminded me of a travelling shop in west Cavan long ago. And they brought me exotic stories about monastic life in Belarus, and their battered van of icons was a symbol of absurd hope in the secular world I lived in.

It was their stories that I loved. I sat for hours listening to them recounting tales of love and death, and everyday saints in a faraway monastery covered in snow. The truth was not the issue. But the way they told it gladdened my heart.

Our house was small, but we had access to an apartment in Carrick-on-Shannon where we assured them they could stay and enjoy complete privacy.

And they agreed to stay, and the apartment was given over to them for a week, so that they could come and go as they pleased.

Under their saintly veils, and inside their starch and formal skirts, their hearts were as vibrant and modern as any young person of that age; they had an interest in Irish music, pop bands, Netflix and iPhones.

One of them had fluent English and one of them had so little that she smiled constantly in a state of confusion.

They hugged us and laughed and straightened their veils and rolled up their sleeves and wanted to do the washing-up after meals although we wouldn't let them.

And they spoke about Dostoyevsky and a book about monks called *Everyday Saints*, which they said was a best-seller in Russia, and one of them played the tin whistle and said she studied music, and she sang the Greek hymn to the Virgin Mary, 'Agni Parthene', and when the meal was ready

I sat at the head of the table and, having totally lost the run of myself, invited them to say a prayer.

I bowed my head and allowed the delicious Russian prayers to flow over me.

I found videos of the Saint Elisabeth monastery in Minsk. I listened to their choir singing. I watched documentaries that a Russian television station had made about a famous musician who directed their choirs. I played chanting monks from Valeem for them, with them. And it was as if all my prayers in Warsaw had found their fullness.

One night I dreamed of snow, and Moscow, and a monastery in Minsk. In the morning I googled the monastery. I wanted to visit it.

257

And when I wasn't dreaming my way into a monastery in Minsk I was slipping back into depression. Except that this time it felt my body was dragging me back. And I was fighting against it. It's usually the heart that sinks first into melancholy, and the body follows. But this time my heart was on fire with excitement, and it was the body that seemed strangely and disturbingly leaden.

But one way or another, I was in the dark. The shadows grew around me. I knew I was in the middle of a struggle. I just didn't know how ferociously my heart was struggling to pump blood to every remote region of my body, and how close it was to failure.

After a few days the women phoned us from the apartment and said they were heading west; Dimitri would drive them to Castlebar and other western targets to flog their holy pictures.

'Feel free to come back and use the apartment anytime you wish,' I said.

Two days later they returned and again we stood around the dining table, hugging them like we were their favourite uncle and auntie, and they prayed again for a blessing on the food, and I told them I had been looking at their monastery on Google, and I had watched videos of their Christmas services, and how the monastery looked so beautiful in the snow.

'Then you must come for Christmas,' one of them said.

Was it a joke? I wasn't sure. I waited before reacting. She was gazing straight at me. Blue-eyed, and honest, and without irony.

'Yes,' she said again, 'you must come for Christmas. It is a beautiful time to visit our monastery.'

'I would love to,' I said, taking a quick look at the beloved.

'Then yes,' they said, 'you must come. It is possible.'

'No, no,' I said, picking up the word. 'No, I don't actually think it is really possible,'

I glanced at the beloved.

'Don't look at me,' she joked.

'But it might be very difficult to get a visa for Belarus,' I conjectured, edging closer to the prize. 'And maybe that time of year would not be good.'

The one who had so little English suddenly seemed as if she had been following the conversation quite well.

'Almost everything is possible,' she said quietly, with her eyes on the table as if she were speaking to herself.

'What about visas?' I asked, moving now to clinch the prize.

'If you land by plane at the international airport,' she said, 'it is not a problem. You get the visa when you arrive.'

That was in mid-November. Before the end of the month I had booked a ticket to travel from Dublin to Minsk, via Germany, on 4 January.

I emailed the brother in charge of hospitality at the monastery and received a welcome reply saying that they would not charge me for my stay, and that they would reserve a room for seven nights.

The nights in late November were getting darker. The winter was enfolding us. The damp cloak of depression had disabled me every morning from the time I woke, and I woke exhausted. But again it felt more a physical exhaustion than trouble of the heart.

My heart was already in the snow of Belarus, among the Christmas trees and the golden light of icons burnished by flickering candles.

I had hope in the dark winter for the first time in a few years. I had something to look forward to.

Our own simple Christmas was always joyful. We lit up a tree. We placed the same crib beneath it, as we did every winter for twenty-five years. We bought a lot of wine, and usually got a friend to make delicious Indian dishes for Christmas Day.

The family gathered – the daughter and the boy child and his wife. We would sit around for two days and nights to mark the darkest moment of the winter with that shared food and wine, and feel reinvigorated for the new year. It was ritual, without anything overtly religious about it.

But when that was over, I could slip away for another Christmas, a second, Orthodox Christmas, in the snow; a banquet of light, incense and chanting in the heart of an ancient Orthodox convent. The very thought of it brought me close to ecstasy.

The death of strangers

aving the sisters as our guests for a week had been a
delight, even though they came and went, and had
lots of space to get on with their own affairs. But
they came to us for evening meals on a number of occasions
during the week and those were the climactic moments; and
what crowned everything, like a moment of transfiguration,
was when they mentioned Colmcille.

It was on the second evening, as we finished supper, the sister
with good English was explaining how large their monastery was,
and how their choirs travelled around Europe giving recitals,
and how one of their nuns had been married to a composer who
died tragically, and triggered her wish to enter the convent.

'Music,' she said, 'is the most important thing in our
monastery.'

'And I saw on your website that you also have a workshop
making icons,' I said.

'Oh yes,' she said, 'we have, eh, eight hundred people in
the workshop, making icons of all saints.'

And it was clear she wanted to be inclusive: 'Including the Irish saints,' she added.

Which surprised me.

'Yes,' she said. 'We write icons of Patrick, and to us he is Saint Patrick, and we can also write icons of other saints.'

'Brigid,' the silent sister whispered.

'And Finbarr. And Aideen.'

They had done their homework. She was reaching for other names. And the name I wanted to hear was Colmcille. So I said it.

262   'Colmcille?'

But no.

'Who is this?' she asked.

She didn't know. I was flattened.

But then the silent one spoke up again. 'Columba,' she said. 'We call him Saint Columba of Scotland.'

'Ah yes,' her companion said. 'Columba. Of course.'

'What. Did. Eh. You. Call. Heem?' the silent one inquired.

'Colmcille,' I said.

'Saint Colmcille,' she whispered, 'pray for us.'

That house in Glencolmcille felt like it was mine.

For a while we all had our heads bowed – the sisters, the beloved and me – as we all searched our own little Google screens to find icons of the famous Donegal man. We passed the phones around, examining this or that variation of the saint.

I was so far gone with delusions of my exceptionality, my ludicrous liaison with a divine being, that had I fallen down at that moment with heart failure I might have whispered on my last breath that it was a joy to die in the certain knowledge that Colmcille would escort me to heaven because he had appeared to me on an iPhone.

'Could you make an icon of Columba?' I wondered.

'Yes,' she said. 'If you like.'

I pointed to an image on her iPhone. 'I would like this one,' I said.

The icon I found depicted the monk at his desk, writing a poem. He had grey hair. Sandalled feet. He had a desk and a pen and ink, and he was writing. In a sense I saw it as an icon of the saint as poet.

263

If I ordered it, and they could write it, make it, within two months, then it made more sense of my planned Christmas holiday.

'I can collect the icon when I visit your monastery for Christmas,' I said, hugely inflated by how the pattern and jigsaw of life was fitting into place in a manner that so pleased me.

Little did I know that everything was about to be destroyed; all my time in Warsaw, all my little churches, oratories, icons and sanctuaries of the heart, with all their bells and whistles and holy candles, and all my airy saints and glens and cottages and edifices of fantasy were about to fall.

All my wasted time, alone, my universe, my everything. It was all about to crumble.

But even after the holy sisters had come and gone, there were more deaths at the end of November, and I felt the quiet burden of them as if they were lead inside my heart. Sometimes I could detect a gentle pain on the in-breath. A tightness as I sucked up the oxygen.

The death of a stranger I didn't know, but whose tragic end was related to me casually on the apron of a filling station, stuck in my craw for days.

He was a local boy, I was told, who died by his own hand in the farm shed after a few hours in the pub. I was at a petrol station in Carrick-on-Shannon when I met a friend in a black suit. He was returning from the funeral.

'We were burying the nephew,' he said.

'What happened?' I wondered.

'He went into the shed one night,' the man declared. I nodded because we all know what can happen to a young man, alone in a shed.

'He texted his friends,' the man said, 'and told them to bring the guards. But he was dead when they got there, and his neck was badly marked with his fingernails. He must have regretted it at the last moment.'

I listened.

I didn't say anything, because there is a grief that words cannot soften, and a pain that no story can cure.

'There's too much rain and forestry in Leitrim,' he said as we parted. 'No wonder the graveyards are full of young men.'

I walked away as numb as if someone had told me I might be next.

Snow

On the first week of December 2018 I was in the National Concert Hall for a recording of *Sunday Miscellany*. I stood aloof from the other readers in the green room behind the stage.

Joe Duffy was there. Catriona Crowe. Eileen Battersby.

I felt tired. I even resented being there because I had three shows of my own that week. Three nights of standing on stage for ninety minutes reading from my book.

Why did I agree to do this?

I felt, well, it's only ten minutes on stage. That shouldn't be too much bother.

But when the day comes it's always the same. It's never ten minutes. It's a full day. Travelling, finding a hotel for the night, going to the venue to do a sound check at 5 p.m. which then doesn't really happen until 7.30 p.m. And then I stand around the wings for the entire show.

I might not be on stage all the time, but I'm on edge.

Yet I wanted to be there because the piece I was reading mattered to me. I had been through a strange and lonely year. I had spent winter alone in Warsaw, and I returned at the height of summer for a further month. My sixty-fifth year felt like a turning point. And I had written a piece that summed it up. A synopsis of that dark despondency and grim sense of mortality that was soaking into my heart like ink into blotting paper.

'I was in Warsaw last winter,' I told the audience …

266

… and every day I waited for snow. But none came. Rain came. Wind. And sleet.

Sometimes flakes, falling like salt that barely coated the pavement.

But all the while I longed for more.

At night the cars parked below my eighth-floor window turned white in the frost, but by dawn the rain had washed them clean.

I worried about this lack of snow. An old lady in the next apartment worried. Every morning we met in the escalator and we worried together.

'No snow today,' I said.

'Climate heating,' she said. 'My grandchildren are sad; last month at Christmas they had no snow.'

I was snug in bed one night, when my nose detected something. I didn't turn on a light because the city beyond my balcony glowed with neon lights. I looked out.

The traffic on John Paul Avenue and the neon signs near Arkadia shopping centre were wrapped in a blizzard; and a million white flakes enveloped the apartment blocks around me.

On the quadrangle below, a patch of grass was already white, and by the print of boots I knew the snow was already thick.

It was after midnight but children had been taken from their beds, and were tobogganing down a slope as their fathers in anoraks and hoodies smoked and chatted under the streetlamps.

267

'It was lovely to see the snow last night,' I said to the old lady the next day.

'Oh yes,' she said.

But she seemed broken-hearted, as she pressed the escalator button.

'The snows are melting,' she said, 'all the time.'

I associate snow with Russian literature. In novels by Tolstoy or Pasternak, characters are always dying in the snow, or running after trams in the snow, or just waiting for the train to arrive late from Saint Petersburg.

Snow is a remarkable ingredient in storytelling. It hides the entire world. It allows us to conjure invisible things, like secrets of the heart that remain hidden from view.

A young friend of mine from Belarus once explained to me what the difference is between East and West.

'In Russia,' she said, 'the most real things are on the

inside. But in the West, you live always on the outside.'

The Russian poet Irina Ratushinskaya lived on the inside. She hadn't much choice.

She spent four winters in a prison cell during the 1980s. She was confined to a tiny hut, where the freezing ice soaked into her bones and broke her health.

In that solitary confinement she was deprived of pen or paper for fear she might write subversive poems against the state.

So she scribbled away on a bar of soap with a matchstick. Then she would smooth the soap and begin another verse. Verse by verse she composed and memorised over 400 poems, keeping them hidden in her heart until she was released.

She died in 2017. She was sixty-three. All she wanted in the end was to die at home in her husband's arms. And so she did. Passing away with a smile on her lips. Because she did not believe in death. Perhaps she had a soul, hidden behind her smile, which flew to some invisible heaven on her last breath.

At least that's the way I like to imagine it, with the curve of poetry in the bleak shape of any death.

I remember standing at my mother's grave one snowy Christmas morning and sensing that she was not lying in the clay before me, but in the air, invisible and just beyond my fingertips.

Snow makes it easy to believe in the invisible. And in the possibility of a human soul. A kind of deeper hidden self, like a mountain obscured in a blizzard.

But like the woman in the escalator, the lack of snow worries me. In scientific terms we may end up living in a world without snow. But it is snow as a metaphor that matters most to me. And that is in danger.

I was coming to my overall point. And I took a breath here as I read.

I felt pain in my chest.

The audience were silent. You could hear a pin drop. I knew that I had delivered the most intense and personal essay for *Sunday Miscellany* that I had ever written. Looking out at the sea of faces beyond the microphone, I felt dizzy and the faces blurred. They were waiting for me to continue. But they almost drew me to tears.

The script on the podium beneath the microphone continued with the word 'we'.

But I knew that little pronoun was a mask for more personal feelings. So as I read, I edited the text, changing the personal pronoun into the singular, to bare my soul completely with the audience.

Why wouldn't I?

It felt for certain like the last *Sunday Miscellany* I would ever do.

'I exist,' I declared to the audience …

… on the surface of things. I wallow in the visible. I seek only the reality of tangible objects. I have forgotten the very

soul that breathes inside me. The soul that can endure the fiercest blizzard. The hidden heart, where poetry gets born, even though we be, for now, in a prison cell.

When I finished, I staggered back into the wings, where Eileen Battersby was waiting for her moment on stage. She looked at me, and I at her. We worked for the same newspaper but had never been properly introduced. I wanted to say something but I couldn't. I was too frazzled. And there was something in her eyes too. So I just nodded, whispered a brief hello and went out into the corridor.

Then I became deliciously invisible as I sat in a corner, close to where some musicians from the orchestra were waiting for their moment on stage.

I didn't know why my heart had turned so black. It wasn't depression. It was like the tiredness that comes at the end of a party. When it's over. When you want to go home. Four-in-the-morning tiredness. When you have walked far enough and you want to lie down.

I had said hello to Eileen Battersby because she too worked with *The Irish Times*, and since I never actually visited the IT building in Dublin, I had never actually met her. I wanted to chat with her. When her piece was over and she came down the corridor towards the green room I congratulated her on it. And then said who I was.

'Oh, I know you,' she said, smiling, and for a second it felt like we might have lots to talk about. But then the darkness descended on me again.

What's the point in talking to anyone, a voice whispered inside me. So I left it at that. And I left the building.

Which I regretted deeply some weeks later when Eileen was killed in a car accident.

Life can be fragile. The ice is thin. And I felt I too was on the verge of catastrophe.

The following night I was on stage in Bray, and the night after that in Blanchardstown. But after the Blanchardstown gig I walked back to the hotel with a pain in my chest, which had persisted since that morning, and it endured all through the night, until sometime after 9 a.m., in room 725 of the four-star Crown Plaza Hotel, when I had a heart attack.

Poached eggs

phoned 999 from my hotel room. I asked for an ambulance and gave my room number. But I forgot to alert hotel reception. So when the ambulance arrived the hotel staff knew nothing about it.

The paramedics told the receptionist that the call came from room 725.

The phone beside my bed rang.

'Good morning, sir,' the receptionist said, 'did you order an ambulance?'

I wanted to say, 'No, I ordered poached eggs.' But the tension at the reception desk might have been exacerbated if I tried to be funny.

The hotel manager wanted to find out what had happened in room 725 so he came up in the lift with the paramedics.

Moments later two young men in high-visibility jackets were standing over me, with aspirin, and other tablets, as I lay stretched on the bed.

The hotel manager remained at the door.

A mother and daughter pushing suitcases along the corridor stopped to gawk, until the manager discreetly closed the door.

One paramedic handed me a tablet. 'Don't swallow,' he said. 'Chew it first.'

I chewed like a dog with a morsel of bone. For some reason I was talking to myself.

'Apparently Robert Lowell died in a taxi,' I declared.

The paramedics didn't hear me. They wheeled me to the lift, down to the foyer and out the front door, into the back of an ambulance.

I've seen a lot of ambulances taking people away, from supermarkets, public houses and hotel foyers. It's always the same; the ambulance arrives and the blue light spins. Another casualty of life is wheeled to the waiting vehicle. The back doors are slammed shut and the ambulance screams away into the traffic. Now it was me in the lead role.

'I'm sorry to have bothered you,' I said to the paramedic, as we sped through the traffic lights and criss-crossed Blanchardstown. 'It was just indigestion.'

He smiled. 'We'll be there in a minute,' he said.

And we were; and for a few hours my life, as they say, was in their hands.

I remember waking in the night and seeing a nurse staring into my eyes.

'Are you OK?' she asked.

Her oval face and brown skin were lit by almond eyes.

274

'Where are you from?' I wondered.

'India,' she said.

'Am I dreaming?' I wondered.

'No,' she said. 'You just had a heart attack. Tomorrow the consultant will put in a stent. There is nothing to worry about.'

Which wasn't exactly true. I was worried that I might need to use the toilet.

'We can get you a bed pan if you need one,' she said. I closed my eyes and tried to sleep.

The stent was inserted the following afternoon; a near-miraculous procedure whereby a scaffolding is placed inside the clogged artery to allow a free flow of blood.

The procedure was executed with precision by the dexterous hands and eyes of a heart surgeon who spoke gently to me as I lay on the table before him. For some reason I got the notion that he might be from Kerry, and so, considering the masterful precision and dexterity of that county's champions in both football and dancing, it seemed reasonable to believe that a Kerryman would excel equally well at heart surgery.

I tried without success to engage him in conversation about Skellig Michael, Orthodox monks and Kerry dancers, as I lay flat and almost naked on his table, with a gigantic television screen above my head and various people in eggshell blue uniforms moving about the operating room.

When I was young a heart attack often signified sudden death somewhere casual, like the ninth green of the golf

275

links. And surgery, when required, left scars from the neck to the bellybutton. Men wandered the hospital corridors in dressing gowns with despairing faces and in dreadful pain.

So I was lucky. And I was full with gratitude. I wanted to hug the entire hospital and everyone in it. It was 9 December.

The virgin in the crib

On 8 December when I was a child, everything closed down and we all went to Dublin in an Austin A40. It was the only possibility of meeting Santa face-to-face and whispering into his ear the thing I wanted for Christmas.

The postal service in Cavan was a pure cod. That's what my mother often said when the Christmas cards arrived on the second day of January.

I used to drop my letter for Santa in the post box outside the Market Square, but that was usually a day or two before Christmas Eve, so no one could convince me that a letter with no address would ever get to the North Pole.

Dublin was the only chance to get a word in Santa's ear, just after Mammy had completed her quest for the fabled Hafner's sausages and white puddings that were so essential in her turkey stuffing.

After that we'd head over to see the fat man with the white beard in his red dressing gown in Arnotts. Mammy seemed to swallow the performance hook, line and sinker so I usually ignored the fact that Santa's arse could hardly contain itself on the chair he was sitting on, never mind trying to manoeuvre it down our chimney, even if there wasn't a coal fire burning in the grate below.

Simply put, this was a fake Santa, no matter how many adults believed him. But I didn't want to be the one to tell Mammy.

In my letter that year I said I wanted a bicycle. I was too old for teddies. So I asked for a Raleigh. But in the ear of the beardy man at Santa's grotto I opted for the teddy; I told him I'd love another cuddly bear.

It was a bicycle that arrived in the yard on Christmas morning, certain proof, my mother asserted, that Santa had received the letter.

'He couldn't get it down the chimney,' Mammy explained. Although I noticed that he couldn't manage to tear the price docket off the front wheel either.

After that I was sceptical about Christmas for a few years. But when I was thirteen I found some kind of enlightenment.

That year I carried the Virgin Mary, with the aid of another altar boy, from the sacristy, across the sanctuary to the crib. She was as big as either of us. But when we saw Mary Brady, a skinny girl in a Loreto uniform, lighting a candle, my friend said, 'There's that one from Stradone.'

And when I turned to gawk, I slipped on the sanctuary steps and the Mother of God went skidding across the marble floor.

Fortunately there were only a few scratches on her fingers so we picked her up and got her into the manger with her eyes focused on the baby Jesus and her hands joined.

When the people gathered around the crib that Christmas night I was terrified someone might notice the damage.

The bishop, an old man with enormous white eyebrows, gave the crib a skite of holy water. Drops landed on Mary's face and I feared the congregation would see the scratches on her fingers due to our wanton sexual desires for Mary Brady.

I knew it was only a statue. And a few scratches to the fingers of a porcelain virgin was hardly going to alter the direction of the universe.

And yet all the people blessed themselves and prayed with closed eyes – Hail Mary, full of Grace – as if she were of flesh and blood, and kneeling there before them in the straw.

The real Mary, I concluded, must indeed be hiding behind the image, and orchestrating the universe's pulse to suit me. And the real Christ must be hidden behind the garish baby in the straw.

The light was hidden in the darkness, as Old-Bishop-Eyebrows said in his sermon.

But my real enlightenment related to Santa.

I concluded that was real.

And perhaps behind the sham of gaudy rituals, in which men with white curly beards and red dressing gowns posed for pictures with frightened infants, there might be a deeper secret – that of infinite generosity.

All the gaudy Santas in department stores and village halls were only there to comfort adults, who could no longer accept the possibility of the invisible made visible.

The white-haired man

We camped in the van for two nights. One night was spent on the cliffs above Glencolmcille and one night in the sand dunes near the airport outside the village of Annagry.

Now we had checked into the Caisleáin Óir Hotel. And it was good to lie in a cosy bed with the beloved resting beside me, checking her iPad, as I stared at the end of *Newsnight* on BBC.

'I'm going to bed,' she declared. 'I'm tired.'

'It's early yet,' I said. 'It's only eleven o'clock.'

'You go back down if you like,' she suggested.

So down I went and sat by the window in the bar for a short while, looking out at the car park and the camper van in the corner. I had spent 5,500 euros on that little black bus, I thought, and here we are checking into a hotel. But I suppose we needed a rest.

Then a short little man with a bald head, carrying a shopping bag, sat down beside me.

The waitress came towards us.

'You're here for the scenery, are you?' he said to me.

'I'm just on holidays,' I said.

'I'm just back from Aranmore,' he declared.

He didn't really care whether I was on holidays or landed recently from Mars. He just wanted conversation in that way that country people who live alone relish strangers in a public house.

'There was a party on the island last night,' he said. 'For a girleen that would be a daughter of a man I worked with for years in London. She was thirty so all the young people went in to the island and drank far too much and this morning they were still at it.

'In the pier bar. All lined up, young rascals, like whippets, and them guzzling drink, and outside around a table in the sunshine all the girls were on the vodka and gin, like new lambs guzzling from the tit of a bottle, and them singing.

'And when we were getting into the ferry to come back out from the island this morning they were still at it. With bottles and cans and them all lunging this way and that on the top deck of the ferry. What I was asking myself is what will they do when they get to Burtonport. Will they continue, or will they get into cars and go kill themselves.'

'They're good singers in Donegal,' I suggested.

'They're agreeable enough,' he admitted, 'but they're wicked bad at the driving.'

'What do you think of Daniel O'Donnell?' I wondered.

The folds of flesh around his eyes moved liked a waking

282

walrus, and eyeballs blue as the sea swung towards me, holding me in a firm, interrogative grip.

Then he touched my elbow and confided in me, whispering, 'Daniel had an uncle was a far better singer.'

He muttered it under his breath, as if he feared the walls might hear his blasphemy.

A car arrived outside at high speed, leaving tyre marks at the bend outside the hotel before coming to a halt.

'God take care of us all,' the man muttered. 'And me looking for a lift to Gaoth Dobhair, but sure it's only up the road. I might be safer walking.'

283

The young man who had just skidded his car into the car park arrived at the door of the lounge, looked about, recognised my companion and sauntered over.

'That's me taxi,' the man said. 'So now, enjoy your drink.'

And he hopped up with his bag, and went out the door, waddling obediently behind his driver.

My walk with the beloved earlier that evening to the sea, and the wine and sirloin steak, had tired me. And I was tempted to go back upstairs to bed. But I love the open-hearted conversation in country pubs, how easy it is to blend in and how people will sit and talk to any stranger, as if they had known them for years.

So I decided to hang on for another solitary drink.

When we were young, the beloved and I cycled around Donegal. We loved the beaches. We'd lie on the strand just to hear the waves thunder as the ocean approached. Now I experience that same vulnerability everywhere. Because old people don't need the sea to feel powerless. Fragility grows with the years, and something unnameable roars at me, even in the fury of rush-hour traffic, like an ocean that must be faced eventually.

It's not just in Warsaw that I walked.

I walked everywhere. At least before the heart attack.

In Paris I used to walk from the 6th arrondissement where I stayed in the Centre Irlandais, writing a book called *Bird in the Snow*, down the hill into town, past Notre Dame, through Saint-Denis and up to the Sacred Heart. I loved the cool sanctity of Notre Dame, followed by all the doorways in Saint-Denis where the whores stood trying to catch my eye. I loved the laundromats full of North African women who would fold their arms and stare at me, before I climbed the steps up to the majestic Church of the Sacred Heart and listen to nuns in starched white habits singing vespers in the late afternoon.

And I walked on Banna Strand.

Along the Cliffs of Moher.

And up and down Manhattan.

Berlin. Naples.

And the lovely towns of south Ulster, Dundalk, Monaghan, Cavan, Enniskillen, Fivemiletown and Ballyshannon.

And all the other little towns in Ireland, where I did book-readings on tour.

I walked up Sliabh Liag twice, and Earagail when I was a teenager, and stood at the very summit holding onto the iron railings as I looked across the entire county, and then up Croagh Patrick with expensive glasses and back down without them.

Ireland is beautiful, and the part of it that I love most is the Atlantic coast, but in all the two thousand miles of Wild Atlantic Way there was one spot sweeter for me at that time than all the rest.

And that was Glencolmcille.

I had dreamed of living there. I had dreamed of the saint there, like a guide from heaven.

But it all collapsed in a heart attack, and I had to call the auctioneer and ask for my money back, and explain the catastrophe. I had to get the doctor to write a note, to whom it may concern, that I had an acute coronary attack, and I sent it to the airline company to get that money back too, because the flight had been insured.

285

And in the end, though we could not afford a house, nonetheless with a camper van we reached the ocean easily and we lay on the edge of the world.

We had stood on a cliff above Glencolmcille forty-eight hours earlier. The beloved had slept and I'd got out before dawn and walked a few metres to urinate, and to hear the ocean roar.

It had been sufficient proof for me that we had been guided to our destination.

I would go no more a-roving, a-wandering in the night. I would search no more for meaning. And I would not hunger again for exotic churches in far-off worlds.

I was home.

I had an icon in the van to prove it, the same icon which I commissioned from the sisters, and which their workshop had crafted during the winter, and which they brought back to Ireland with them in March since I could not make the journey to Minsk for Christmas on account of the illness.

I imagined Colmcille the writer as a difficult young man who stirred trouble everywhere, until he found peace on the island of Iona. I imagined him as a wise middle-aged artist who wrote poems and fathered elaborate masterpieces like the Book of Kells. And I imagined him in old age, a white-haired abbot of orthodox Christianity who fell down dead from heart failure, quietly, one morning as he said preparatory prayers before the Divine Liturgies of the day in the main chapel in Iona.

In the icon made in the Saint Elisabeth Convent in Minsk an old white-haired man sits at his desk with pen and ink, and in his hand is a scroll and on the scroll are the words of a poem he is composing.

'That I might see the heavy waves, as they sing their music to the Heavenly Father.' It is written in Gaelic and the words are directly from the pen of the saint.

The previous day I too had seen the waves swell and crash against the rocks and cliffs of Malin More, singing to the great Atlantic sky, just below where the van was camped; and on the morrow I would step further out of time and into that silence which lies at the heart of all ritual, as I joined other pilgrims on the long, winding path around the holy stones of Glencolmcille.

There were still a few people drinking in the bar, although the family groups had all gone. It was after midnight and the barman was tired.

He was only a boy.

Earlier Liverpool had won on the big screen and two married women were discussing the game as they sat on high stools. It was close to closing time so I knew the barman would not come down to my table.

Instead I went to the bar, ordered a drink and used the moment as an excuse to sit not far from the women.

Unfortunately I didn't notice a man with an English accent and an overbearing manner at the bar lecturing the barman on how to make a proper martini.

287

The two women ordered gin. The barman fixed them little measures of Gunpowder mixed with tonic and loads of ice in long, slim blue glasses.

'Those are not the correct glasses,' the Englishman declared. 'You've got to serve gin in a gin glass.'

The boy behind the bar shrugged. 'Those are the glasses that come with the gin. The sales rep gave them to us.'

'Oh well, the rep is wrong, isn't he?'

'Well, they make the gin,' the boy insisted.

And I'm thinking, fair play to you, young fellow. You won't be put down.

'Then the gin company has got it wrong. What gin is it anyway?' And he spelled out the name. 'Drum. Shan. Bo. Where the fuck is Drum-shan-bo?' he asked.

I was thinking I must be careful here and keep me mouth shut at all costs. Because I'm from Drumshanbo. But I said nothing.

I said nothing, that is, until he came over to me. He had a formidable belly and I felt like telling him that it might be no harm to have his heart checked.

'Them big bellies is fierce dangerous, sir,' I said, joking.

But he didn't hear me. 'Wot you drinking?' he wanted to know.

'I'd prefer to stay on my own, sir,' I confessed.

'Rory, give us a drink here.' He turned to the ladies. 'Ladies,' he said, 'wot you drinking?'

288 The women were sipping from the long blue glasses. 'Gin,' they replied, daring him to get them another one.

But he said, 'Jesus fucking Christ,' because he had noticed they were sucking Mikado biscuits that had been left on the bar counter on someone else's tray. 'Jesus fucking Christ, girls, what are you DOING?'

'Biscuits,' one of them said.

'You can't fucking eat biscuits with gin. It's not fucking right.'

'We can do what we like,' one of them said.

He examined the packet of biscuits on the counter. 'Mikado,' he said. 'Mick-ah-do,' he repeated with derision. 'Do you realise,' he declared, 'that Mikado are the gayest fucking biscuit on the planet? I mean, pardon my French, and I've nothing against gay people, live and let live is wot I say, but fuck it, ladies. You. Can't. Be. Serious.'

The boy behind the bar turned up the volume of the big screen on the wall. A sports programme was playing highlights of the match and showing clips from the press conference afterwards. The manager of Liverpool was on screen talking to the press about the great win they had just had. And then he started crying, and the Englishman was irritated because the intrusion had interrupted his dramatic move on the ladies.

'Turn that down,' he said to the barman, 'we saw that earlier.'

'It's Liverpool,' the barman retorted, and turned it slightly louder.

The ladies swivelled on their high stools away from the man to watch the interview.

'Why is he crying?' one of the women asked the other.

''Cos he's foreign,' the man said. 'Can't stand that guy,' he added. 'Knows nothing about football.'

The women had turned their arses to him now, settling into their gin, and I had my head down with the phone stuck almost up my nose so he wouldn't bother me as an alternative source of conversation.

But then he came. I couldn't ignore him. He leaned his elbow onto the bar beside me and stared at the side of my head until I paid attention.

English people used to be invisible before Brexit. Their accents were melodious in the air, like visiting birds in summertime. They were part of every community in the country, solidly contributing to social life.

Visitors from England in summer time were usually viewed as close cultural relations. In fact, many visitors from England were actually Irish people who had been forced to emigrate, picked up English accents and returned home every summer to keep their children conscious of where they came from.

In any vibrant country parish you'd often hear English accents at public meetings speaking about tidy towns issues, or Special Olympics, or organising street collections for some charity. They rarely joined drama societies, which I suppose is a particularly native kind of madness, but they loved being part of civic society.

In Leitrim they grew vegetables in lonely places; they had lovely voices, and enthusiasms for Radio 4, and often displayed keen moral sensibilities about ecological and economic issues that far outpaced the ethical development of country people driven by self-interest.

And all the English people I ever knew have been polite and charming and I'd cross the Irish Sea in a canoe just to hear the crisp precision with which they use the English language.

But Brexit changed everything.

The two women had been in the lounge earlier with their children and partners, and their partners had gone to bed with the children. The Englishman hadn't been observing much, or he wouldn't have tried to chat up two married women whose children and husbands were just upstairs.

And he didn't succeed with me either. My nose was in the phone. He tried one more time to raise a conversation.

'Where you from?' he said, squinting at me like he had me sussed as a Russian spy.

'Drumshanbo,' I said, with as much dignity and condescension as I could muster.

When he was gone Rory turned off the television, the women turned to me, and we all had one last drink for the road, although nobody was going anywhere.

'That Gunpowder stuff is good,' one of them remarked.

'It is,' I agreed. As proud as if I had bottled it myself.

Enjoy yourself,
it's later than you think

But what could be better than to lie in a lovely double bed with the beloved, in the Caisleáin Óir Hotel on a fine June morning.

With a view of the sea from the window.

I was no stranger to this coastline. I knew its spring tides, its little waves lapping and slapping up against the stone walls on the roadside.

Not only did I first find love with a boy in a bunk bed two miles away when I was in the Gaeltacht and still in primary school, but I got my first kiss from a girl on a stone wall in Aranmore two years later when I was in another Gaeltacht summer school. And even after I resigned from the church it was to the coast of Donegal I went, a few years later, to heal the wounds that had been opened by my flirtation with priestly life.

On that occasion I lived in Braade, a townland overlooking the airport at Carrickfinn, and I spent a winter marching up and down the beach and along the sand dunes in the roaring wind.

And would cycle in and out to Annagry, labouring through the wind like someone who had failed, carrying a burden so heavy in my heart that I might as well have had my mother on the back of the bike.

I walked the road that winter as the spray drifted in ghostly clouds across the walls and pelted the windows of the hotel, and the gable of the chapel and the headstones in the nearby graveyard.

And now my lovely black van was there at the edge of the car park. At the rim of the ocean.

294   I could have sat there all morning, thinking about the past, and Donegal, and the future, the next few hours and what special wonders might be waiting for us as we made our pilgrimage through Glencolmcille.

And I sat admiring the van – its lovely alloy wheels and its smart black snout and the shining engine grille with the iconic Mercedes logo that Frank Healy recently replaced.

Not that the van was an icon. But the icon of Colmcille, made in Minsk, was sitting in a box, and the box was in a rucksack and the rucksack was hanging on a hook in the little wardrobe inside the van.

I beheld the van as if it were a tabernacle. But I couldn't dally there all morning. Our booking included breakfast, and the dining room would soon be closed so I needed to shower, brush my teeth, put on some clothes and head down for scrambled eggs and smoked salmon.

The beloved was already in the shower.

At another table in the dining room the pilot was finishing his coffee, the sleeves of his white pilot's shirt rolled up, while two cabin crew in green Aer Lingus uniforms buttered their last fingers of toast.

An American woman was making a fuss about the plate on which her poached eggs arrived. Apparently the plate was cold.

I ordered poached eggs too, with smoked salmon. The beloved just had eggs.

I didn't think I would like smoked salmon; it's cold texture wasn't something I would have ordered heretofore, but I was trying to eat more heart-friendly foods.

295

I noticed people at other tables using slices of lemon on their fish, so I called for a little lemon and squeezed it over the salmon and to my astonishment it tasted delicious.

I dipped the salmon in the eggs too, and they were much improved and livelier to taste from contact with the bitter fish.

In the hotel foyer two Americans were getting advice from the woman at reception as I passed. The receptionist was suggesting routes they might take along the Wild Atlantic Way. Restaurants they might enjoy. Places associated with Daniel O'Donnell. The airport. Packie Bonner, Ireland's mythic goalkeeper.

Then one of them asked why the hotel was called An Caisleáin Óir. What did it mean?

The receptionist explained how it was the title of a book by a famous writer from the area called Séamus Mac Grianna.

I knew all that. And I knew too that it was Seosamh, the

brother whose bleak life haunted me.

The beloved was still upstairs, checking something about the painter Derek Hill on her iPad, and checkout wasn't until noon.

'I'm just looking at where Derek Hill's house is,' she'd said. 'It would be lovely to drop in there before we head for Glencolmcille.'

So I'd said sure, that would suit, because I wanted to wander across the road and stretch my legs.

I reminded myself that unlike Colmcille, Seosamh Mac Grianna didn't talk to the sea or find equanimity as life went on. He was lost for decades in a Dublin bedsit, with stale milk bottles on the window ledge, blue moulding bread on a shelf and unwashed clothes in heaps behind the door.

He had a mountain of books jumbled up on one single bed, and a second single bed where he slept. Those grim little rooms were not unusual during the thirties or forties in Dublin city, where men endured solitude with no consolations of faith like a monk might be graced with, but only the gritty truths of mid-century Europe, oppressed by authoritarian churches, on the one hand, and the sense that secular life was a hopeless abyss, on the other hand.

I blessed myself with holy water and went inside the church beside the graveyard. I felt nothing. Then I blessed myself again on the way out.

IThere were many white stones in the graveyard and the surname Mac Grianna appeared on many of them. But in the end I could not find his resting place. Although I could hear him.

Whispering.

'Take me with you.'

'No way,' I said. 'This journey is for me and the beloved. I'm not hanging around with hermits or reclusive writers any longer. It's over.'

'It was over for me too,' he whispered back. 'There came a day in 1935 when I knew the well was dry. I would write no more. I couldn't give a damn by then.'

'Yes,' I said, 'I know all that. You stopped writing because you sank into despair.'

'Then my wife died.'

'I know.'

'And my son. All in the one year. It was unbearable.'

'And you were alone, with writer's block. Unable to put pen to paper. It must have been a torment.'

'So take me with you.'

'No. You wouldn't suit Glencolmcille,' I said.

'Colmcille was a writer too,' the shadow said.

Which was true.

'He was a poet,' I said to the shadow. 'But he turned his back on the world for the sake of love. You turned your back on it because you were ill. There's a difference.'

The shadow was gone, and I felt lonely. As they say in Irish, *Tháinig uaigneas orm.*

Uaigneas, a hauntingly beautiful word that comes from *uaig*, a grave.

I remember asking the cardiologist, at the end of my final check-up, how exactly did I get a heart attack. After all is said and done, I exercised, and I wasn't terribly overweight, and I didn't drink to wild excesses.

'We all grow old,' he said, and smiled.

'And is there anything in particular I should do?' I wondered.

'Yes,' he replied. 'Enjoy life. It's later than you think.'

298

Fish and chips,
and the takeaway van

We drove off at noon and stopped in Crolly for fuel. I hopped out to fill the tank with diesel. In the shop I could hear a woman talking to a young girl behind the counter in Irish.

I paid the money.

I wanted a conversation.

'How far is it to Gartan?' I wondered.

'Forty minutes,' the girl behind the counter said.

'We're looking for the Derek Hill Art Gallery,' I explained. And then the other woman joined in, and we all got into a long conversation about the great painter, and how the OPW had renovated the house and how they had a coffee shop with delicious buns.

'And have a great day,' the woman said as I left and the girl behind the counter smiled.

I walked out the door as if on air.

I belonged. I could barely contain myself getting back into the jeep.

Beyond Crolly, we passed Teach Leo, the pub where Enya and the other gifted children of Leo Brennan grew up, sometimes serving in the bar, while their father, a great big stout man with a long nose and a powerful smile, stood in the corner of the lounge, a huge accordion strapped to his shoulders, as he sang out the songs that shaped his children's imaginations.

And then onwards towards the slopes of Earagail as the mountain bog and sky opened up before our van.

We went miles in silence, sometimes only sharing an occasional phrase, like any couple long familiar with the workings of each other's minds.

'This is a pilgrimage for you,' she remarked.

'Yes,' I agreed. 'It is, very much so.'

'It takes me back too,' she said, 'to my childhood.'

'Yes,' I agreed. 'It takes us all back. And I feel grateful to be alive.'

'That's it,' she said.

In Donegal the thread of a human life seems elegantly unimportant compared to the sustained majesty of the earth lying all around like so much debris that some giant had just abandoned – the glinting slate rocks of Earagail and the ocean singing in the distance, and the waves on a dozen beaches, making their song heard through the universe for hundreds of millions of years.

But nothing could make me more lonesome than to stand at the grave of another writer who suffered so much from mental illness. Someone who spent his days, nights, and long autumn afternoons gazing out at the world from a cell in a psychiatric hospital in Letterkenny.

Yet I drove with no shadow in the van. I just imagined him, his bald head out in the ocean as he swam alone and groaned like an old whale. I imagined him walking the roads around Ranafast, knocking on doors and looking through the windows and terrifying the folk within.

Mac Grianna was a kind of embodied darkness. He held in his agony all that I am when I am lonely or melancholic. And even yet he gathers me into his despair and carries me down with him, mythically, if I but allow him.

And like all the dead, he has no more chance to weep. I stood at the grave and whispered a prayer, but in the van I forgot him, because I was just grateful to be alive.

The rocks on the coastline of Donegal are slanted upwards. In some ancient tectonic event one continent crashed into another. The rocks sloping upwards from the sea along the coast bear witness to the event.

Some stones are three hundred million years old. A human life is seventy years or eighty maybe for those who are strong.

And I am sixty-five.

I used to say that kind of stuff to the beloved for years. Then she'd kiss me and we'd go to sleep.

Or sometimes she'd go away.

Sometimes I'd go away.

Then we'd meet again and turn all the same ideas over and over, sitting around coal fires, bonfires, stoves and the embers of many barbecues, drinking a wide variety of alcoholic libations. And sometimes she'd sleep beside me and I would lie awake until the early light of dawn, listening to my Coptic choir singing 'Thou Art the Vineyard'.

I was never uneasy when she was sleeping beside me, as if all the time she were awake and listening. As it says in the Song of Songs, 'My heart turns to you, even in sleep.'

Sometimes among the trees we planted twenty-five years ago I see her, and know we have come full circle.

We hug the shared silence. We acknowledge all the dead, though not as dead, even though we know their dust lies in the ground or has been consumed by the flames of a crematorium. But every time a friend or relation passes away some hidden self that carried them moves deeper into the trees.

We sing our faith like poets utter their verses in the face of night. Not because anything is literally true. But because a poem spoken bears its own and only morality.

We will go down with these songs in our hearts. Singing of eternal life, even though sometimes we don't believe them anymore.

We arrived in Glencolmcille that evening. We parked on a hill overlooking the village, a viewing area with wooden seats and benches, and we went to sleep with the bay and the cliffs all around us, the roofs of the church and the houses below us in the valley.

The pilgrimage began the following afternoon, 9 June, from near the Church of Ireland, just before one o'clock.

It took four hours to complete the path, in the company of a few women and men from the parish, a couple from the South of France, another couple from Dublin and of course the beloved; stopping along the way at various standing stones, and at an old monastic site and a holy well, halfway up the side of a mountain.

The sky was blue above the Church of Ireland, an elegant building shining at the centre of the valley, beside a megalithic tomb and a standing stone from pre-Christian times.

In fact many of the standing stones along the path date back to a prehistoric era, long before Colmcille set his eyes on the waves at Glen Bay.

Etching Christian crosses on standing stones that were already old, even in the sixth century, was an intelligent way of rebranding old truths. Although nowadays it's entirely the memory of Colmcille that haunts the valley.

Halfway up the side of a mountain we stopped at the ruined walls of a church and after circling the building three times, I went inside and lay down on a slab known as *Leabaidh Cholm Cille*.

I turned over three times, and then lifted a handful of clay from beneath the stone, which I'm told can protect a house from fire.

When I was done, the other pilgrims performed the same ritual.

'It's better than house insurance,' a man said, as he folded the black crumbs into an envelope and dropped them gently into his breast pocket.

By the time we got to the holy well I had grown as devout as a Russian nun, and I scooped a full bottle of water from the well to take home with me, promising to distribute it drop by drop to the neighbours.

We all sat down and drank bottled water and ate egg sandwiches and one man told us a story.

'Once upon a time,' he said, 'Colmcille had a stone chalice no bigger than a child's heart, and by drinking from it a person could be cured of anything – the gout within or the gout without, the broken head or the broken heart.'

For centuries the women of Tory Island were the keepers of this chalice, until it was pilfered by fishermen from Scotland. But it only brought bad luck to people who drank from it because it had been stolen, so eventually it was returned to Tory and remained there until the nineteenth century when it vanished again, this time into the delicate hands of a local clergyman, who didn't trust the women of Tory with such a precious relic.

I don't know if the story is true, but I suppose the great thing about religion is that facts always play second fiddle to a myth.

The final standing stone on our journey around the valley had a hole at the top, and in the old days devout pilgrims would gather at it and renounce the world, the flesh and the devil, before looking through the eyehole at the top of the stone in hope that they might see heaven.

There were a lot of rascals with me who wanted to see heaven, but not many takers for renouncing the world.

So I stepped forward, and placed my back to the stone and stretched out my arms three times and spoke my renunciation at the sky with as much fire in my belly as would terrify an infidel. And then I gazed through the eye at the top of the stone and indeed I saw heaven clearly.

Because in every religion, heaven is exactly the same as earth – when your eye has been cured of the jaundiced view.

In the distance the ocean sang as it did when Colmcille stood on the beach and turned his back on Ireland, just so he could contemplate those lovely waves. And the glen around us appeared so peaceful that I knew in my heart it was worth renouncing not just Ireland, but the entire world, for the sake of being there.

And what made it bliss, this narrative of saints and scholars, this cosmology of ghosts that we imagined dancing round us as we walked, what made it blissful was that we were real; humans gathered on that Sunday afternoon with so much irony and so little faith that earlier Christians might have burned us at the stake for being blasphemers.

Four hours later, when the pilgrimage was over, and we had walked the pattern round the hills and said all the prayers that were required, we gathered at the pub, with fish and chips from a takeaway van, and we ate and drank and talked.

One man gave me a remedy for getting ticks out of my arse.

'Just slap a bit of butter on them,' he said. 'It makes them slippery and they'll fall off. That's what we did as children, when we'd come in from the fields.'

But another man had a different remedy.

'Hold the flame of a cigarette lighter close to the tick's backside, and he'll go into reverse middling quick.'

We may have been blasphemers, but we were real to each other. As much as the holy saints were vivid in our imagination, as powerfully as they inhabited our minds and bent our will to their purpose, as a story bends the heart to its conclusions, they bent us out of time, away from any past or future and towards the present moment so that in the end, when we completed the prayers, we were all gathered in the one single and never-ending now.

The beloved and I had found a new way of being alone.

A solitude that both of us inhabited, a solitude that felt like a tent made by God, inside which we were safe.

Although I'd never call the mystery of living in the present moment by that word – God, unless I was dining out with nuns, or people over eighty. And there were none that old in Glencolmcille.

As we drank more pints we became lost in contemplation of one another. The chips were true. The fish was true. And the womenfolk and men who had set out together, come over the black swamp together and climbed to the holy well together, were all true in that moment to each other. And we all agreed that it was only fun, and needed no explaining, and that it might be worth doing again, if the world ever turned around, one more time.

306

Acknowledgements

With thanks to my agent, Marianne Gunn O Connor; Ciara Doorley who edited this book; Bernard and Breda, and all the staff at Hachette Ireland for their continued support.

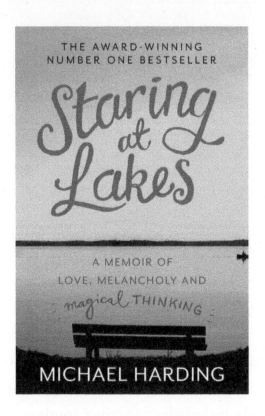

STARING AT LAKES
Bord Gáis Energy Book of the Year 2013

Throughout his life, Michael Harding has lived with a sense of emptiness – through faith, marriage, fatherhood and his career as a writer, a pervading sense of darkness and unease remained.

When he was fifty-eight, he became physically ill and found himself in the grip of a deep melancholy. Here, in this beautifully written memoir, he talks with openness and honesty about his journey: leaving the priesthood when he was in his thirties, settling in Leitrim with his artist wife, the depression that eventually overwhelmed him, and how, ultimately, he found a way out of the dark, by accepting the fragility of love and the importance of now.

Staring at Lakes started out as a book about depression. And then became a story about growing old, the essence of love and marriage – and sitting in cars, staring at lakes.

Also available as an audiobook

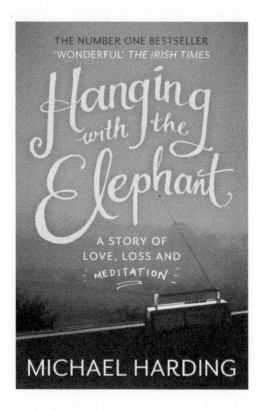

HANGING WITH THE ELEPHANT

'In public or on stage, it's different. I'm fine. I have no bother talking to three hundred people, and sharing my feelings. But when I'm in a room on a one-to-one basis, I get lost. I can never find the right word. Except for that phrase – hold me.'

Michael Harding's wife has departed for a six-week trip, and he has been left alone in their home in Leitrim. Faced with the realities of caring for himself for the first time since his illness two years before, Harding endeavours to tame the 'elephant' – an Asian metaphor for the unruly mind. As he does, he finds himself finally coming to terms with the death of his mother – a loss that has changed him more than he knows.

Funny, searingly honest and profound, *Hanging with the Elephant* pulls back the curtain and reveals what it is really like to be alive.

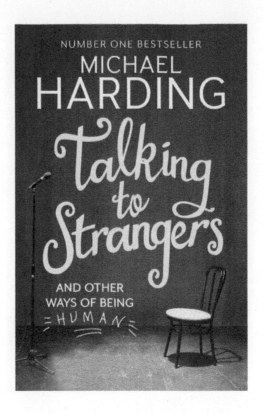

TALKING TO STRANGERS

Too much wine and a casual browse of an airline website – this is how Michael Harding found himself in a strange flat in Bucharest in early January, which set the tone for the rest of that year.

After an intense stint in a high-profile production of *The Field*, Harding returned to the tranquil hills above Lough Allen and started to plan some dramatic changes to his little cottage. Surely an extension would give him a renewed sense of purpose in life as he approached old age.

But as the walls of his home crumbled, so too did his mental health, and he fell, once again, into depression – that great darkness where life feels like nothing more than a waste of time.

And yet, it is in that great darkness that we discover what really makes us human.

Talking to Strangers is a book about love, about the stories we share with others, and the stories we leave behind us.

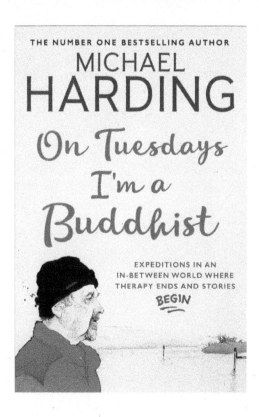

ON TUESDAYS I'M A BUDDHIST

One day in the summer of 2016, Michael Harding's wife brought an unusual gift home from Warsaw. All of a sudden, he found himself falling back into the old religious devotions of an earlier time. The meaning he had found through years of engagement with therapy began to dissolve.

Here, in *On Tuesdays I'm a Buddhist*, Harding examines the search for meaning in life which keeps him fastened to the idea of god.

After many therapy sessions focused on an effort to uncover personal truth, and long solitary months on the road with a one man show, Harding is finally led to an artists' retreat in the shadow of Skellig Michael.

Mixing stories from the road with dispatches from his Irish Times columns, *On Tuesdays I'm a Buddhist* is a spell-binding and powerful book about the human condition, the narratives we weave around the self, and the ultimate bliss of living in the present moment.

An extract from
On Tuesdays I'm a
Buddhist
by Michael Harding
(published in paperback in 2018)

The Client

I was a storyteller originally. As a child, I used to tell myself bedtime stories and I would daydream my way into stories when I was awake. As a teenager, I concocted wild, romantic fantasies about girls on bicycles that could never happen in real life because I was shy and terrified both of the strangeness and familiarity of girls.

But stories and fantasies kept loneliness at bay. I could imagine being with girls. I could imagine holding them. I could imagine what they said and how things always ended with me, the hero, glowing in the light of their adoring gaze.

I was terrified of my teachers too, so I never paid attention in class. Instead, I fell into daydreams. They created a wall between me and whatever was going on in the class.

If I was afraid of shadows in the bedroom at night, I told myself stories. My fear of being alone, isolated and unloved was kept at bay by stories and fairy tales. My anxieties dissolved when I allowed myself to be possessed by a story.

Even now, I'm ashamed to admit, the stories I made up when I was a child were often about my own death – I dreamed that I would die at sixteen. I often imagined my own funeral and all the people in the church talking and chattering about who I was and how they never really understood me but now that I was dead, they could see I was a great hero.

I would imagine the hearse and the service and the burial in the ground. I would imagine the President of Ireland and all the archbishops around the grave. Shots being fired in a gun salute. I was dead, but I had become a hero. That was the story.

And though it was a bleak ritual, it did keep the fear of death at a distance, because it wrapped death up in a story.

My feelings of isolation as a child and my endless anxiety about the imminence of death made me powerless unless I could name it. But when I daydreamed and invented a narrative about accomplishing some heroic deed – fighting for the poor or dying in a hail of bullets, perhaps like the cowboys on the black and white television set – and being buried with military honours while some beautiful young girl sang 'The Streets of Laredo' as my coffin was lowered into the ground by people who, by virtue of my heroic deeds, had come to love me, it was a way of protecting myself from the unease of just being an unlettered nobody, who was stupid, terrified of teachers and enduring life in a constant state of anxiety.

Rather than being powerless in the face of death, I became God in my own little universe of stories. My own little makey-

316

uppy dreamland. And as I grew up, I began to suspect that everyone in the world was the same. We all play out our own fantasies of who we are.

We are all heroes.

We are all in love.

And we all wish to belong in one, single universal story.

And we all still hunger for stories of gods and devils and wonderful deeds. *Game of Thrones* and Harry Potter are narratives we love to inhabit.

We relish the telling of stories. We watch movies with an open heart and with tears in our eyes. We forget we are watching a movie. We become possessed by the truth of the story.

It doesn't matter how well we have seen through the structure of the storytelling or how much we know about archetypal stories or how many workshops on screen-writing classes we have attended. We might have gone to university to get a degree in storytelling or writing, and we might know the back story of every movie character and every heroine in the book. But we have not lost the wonder. We have not lost the hunger for a story. As if all of us, at all times, were made real and true and whole in the stories we tell and the stories we live.

I like *Game of Thrones, House of Cards* and *Star Wars*. And I love the Bible too. I love the stories about Jesus, the songs of Milarepa and the folktales about old monks in the snowy mountains of Tibet hundreds of years ago and the stories that stream onto the pages of a thousand modern novels and the writers groups who share stories and the book-

317

club folk who analyse stories. I especially love the haikus of Chinese poets who died hundreds of years ago, because although the haiku is a brief poem, in every haiku there is a novel and in every novel a person, and in every person there is the possibility of love.

That's the truth, and there isn't a story that was ever told that is not true.

If I tell you a story, we will both be liberated from fear for a short while. Love stories liberating us from the fear of loneliness. Stories of death and heroic destiny liberating us from the fear of our own failures. Protecting us from existential anxiety and from negative emotions. As long as we are telling or listening to a story, we are passing the time wisely.

But we do more than just listen to stories. We live the stories. We shape our lives from stories. Because every one of us is a storyteller. From the time we look in the mirror in the morning and assure ourselves about what we're going to do for the day, what the pattern of our life will be until evening, we are forming stories. And when we lie down to rest on the sofa after a hard day's work, with our eyes half-open, we can't resist yet another story unfolding on the screen of a TV or a laptop.

And what happens between one story and the next? That's the really interesting part. That's the space where we find bliss; where we float sometimes, suspended, and only for a brief moment.

Perhaps only for a few scarce moments in an entire life.

The Sessions

I've talked to my therapist about everything. The weather, the state of the nation, my breakdown in midlife, the death of my mother, my sex life, the significance of cats in my damaged childhood and the enduring loneliness I feel without God. Maybe there will be further issues for us to discuss in future. Things of which I am as yet unconscious and unaware, maybe I'm indulging in cover-ups of things that have yet to come to the surface. Maybe I need more closure. Maybe I am in denial.

Therapy is a strange business. It's like being under investigation for crimes you're not aware of or have not yet committed.

But at its best, it's about words like *opening, trust, listening* and *hope*. The mechanics of it constitute an ongoing dialogue with a skilled guide. It's about sixty minutes every week or every month in a face-to-face meeting between him, the guide, and me, the pilgrim, on a journey towards self-awareness.

I don't go to my therapist consistently, so our sessions happen infrequently. Sometimes, once a year. Sometimes, on a weekly basis for a few months. Sometimes, I don't go near him for years. And this has been going on for most of my adult life.

It began when I was in my twenties. I had friends involved in Gestalt therapy. I had a poster over the bed that said:

I do my thing. You do your thing.

I am not in this world to live up to your expectations. You are not in this world to live up to mine.

If we should find each other, it would be beautiful.

If not, it can't be helped.

Many a night I sat on a beanbag looking up at that poster, hoping it might guide me nakedly to her bed. *That would, indeed, be beautiful*, I thought. Finding her. Imagining myself speaking the words. A phrase I could use in the final moments of seduction, perhaps.

'I am just trying to find you. We are just trying to find each other. Isn't this beautiful?'

But I hated the cool indifference of the final option: *If not, it can't be helped.*

Maybe she was my first real therapist. She was studying sociology and was a good listener with big, blue eyes and a high forehead, and sometimes she would write me letters rather than say something harsh to my face. Eventually, she ended our relationship because she found me too cynical and cold. I think she felt I was too self-obsessed – an observation that time has revealed to be accurate enough. My ego was hurt but in the game we played, she being a kind of proto-therapist and me being the proto-client, it had been a step forward. As the poster said, we didn't meet and it couldn't be helped. But I had learned how the process of therapy worked.

And though I lost a girlfriend, it didn't stop me playing the same games with other girls. Enjoying wonderful sessions. Confessing the riskiest things we could think of. Dicing with shame. Edging our way to unspeakable admissions. Getting erotic charges from the intimacy of truth-telling. Back then, I always got a buzz from the titles of books that might be lying on another person's coffee table or bookshelf.

Gestalt Therapy

I'm OK – You're OK. This Is Me.

By the time I graduated in 1974 with a BA, I had gone to endless weekend courses on gestalt, and transactional analysis. I had done workshops. I had read books. I had visited the primal-scream therapist Jenny James in Donegal. I even visited born-again Christian sects that were governed by middle-aged gurus who used therapy to draw young adults into their own particular narrative of God. I met a load of quacks and crazy people as well as wise and genuine counsellors.

Addiction counsellors.

Guidance counsellors.

I stayed up until dawn at everyone's party, latching on to anyone who would tolerate my narratives of shame, my confessions, who would let me share my secrets with them and test myself as a novice client over a bottle of wine. We sat at kitchen tables with cheap wine until dawn, brain- fucking each other. Believing in each other as true guides and counsellors.

But all those student nights of exhibitionist storytelling amounted to nothing compared to the real thing. The hard, cold eye of a man paid to open you up. I trusted the professional therapist when I met him for the first time. At long last, after a long, solitary childhood, I had someone who listened. And I had been looking for someone to listen.

It was the storyteller in me that found such satisfaction in the confessional narrative of my own personal life. That was crucial. From the very beginning, therapy was only another form of storytelling. Yes, I was an exhibitionist in pain. Yes, I liked showing people where I was wounded. But the satisfaction was in making a story of it all.

And so it was that with a certain amount of enthusiasm, I went alone one day to a semi-detached house on the southside of Dublin, where the therapist's name was engraved on a brass plate outside the black door beneath a Georgian fanlight.

Clearly, there was money in therapy. And I had my wallet in hand to pay.

I was excited to begin the journey. I had a new belonging. I was somebody's client. I had stepped over the threshold and had, at last, arrived in the land of therapy.